"This book is smart and funny and chockful of s[...] beginners and seasoned therapists navigate the t[...] very human mental-health professions. I nodded in agreement, laughed out loud, and sometimes thought 'Gosh, I wish I had known that then.' Highly recommended!"

Michael F. Hoyt, Ph.D., editor of *Therapist Stories of Inspiration, Passion, and Renewal and author of Brief Therapy and Beyond: Stories, Language, Love, Hope, and Time*

"This book addresses issues that may arise as a graduate trainee and early-career psychologist – glitches and snags that you don't read about in text-books or have covered in graduate courses. With humorous anecdotes and engaging stories, Dr. Menard helps the reader come to grips with the fact that we are all fallible and fosters the idea that mistakes are a critical element of personal and professional growth. This book will be a valid-ating resource for anyone wishing to pursue clinical work as a profession."

David J. A. Dozois, Ph.D., CPsych, professor of Psychology and director of the Clinical Psychology Graduate Program, University of Western Ontario

"From managing therapeutic stumbles to gracefully recovering from unex-pected challenges of the early stages of a career in mental health, this book is a beacon of support and an invaluable resource for graduate students and aspiring clinicians alike."

Nawal Mustafa, Ph.D., Neuropsychology and founder of Brain Equilibrium

"This wonderful new book is filled with helpful tips for new therapists. It is personal, candid, and funny, and loaded with important informa-tion that nobody out there seems to talk about. I highly recommend it for anyone who is learning to provide therapy, recently trained therapists, those who supervise therapists in training, and even seasoned therapists."

Martin M. Antony, Ph.D., ABPP, Department of Psychology, Toronto Metropolitan University, Toronto, Ontario, Canada, co-editor, *Handbook of Assessment and Treatment Planning for Psychological Disorders, 3rd ed*

"This is a book for anyone starting out in the field, and anyone who's trying to support anyone starting out in the field. I won't be the first, nor the last, to pick up this book and wonder where it was when I was starting out. Seems a bit unfair that young grad students/interns/early career psychologists get this leg up, when back in MY day we had to flail around, learning everything the HARD way, while beating ourselves up for not knowing what we didn't know before we knew it. Then along comes Dr Dana Menard with her warmth, wisdom, humility, and willingness to use metaphors involving cheap toilet paper (hint: The good stuff is worth the money, people!). It's not only a book with good ideas – I've got plenty of those sitting on my bookshelf. I've even managed to finish a few of them. It's a book with good ideas that's a pleasure to read – and that really is something special."

Dr Jonathan Douglas, Ph.D. CPsych, host of "On Psych: Presented by the Ontario Psychological Association" podcast

"This wise, practical, charming guide is a *must* for anyone who is interested in becoming a therapist, or is in the early stages of their therapist career. But even if you're not on that track, I recommend Dana's book. If you're in therapy and want to get insight into the other side of the couch – or if you're at all interested in mental health and helping others – this is just a great read. It's funny, entertaining, and thought-provoking. It's like Maybe You Should Talk to Someone mixed with What Color is Your Parachute."

A.J. Jacobs, author of *Drop Dead Healthy, The Year of Living Constitutionally and The Know-It-All*

"Lessons from an Early Career Therapist: Managing Mistakes, Missteps, and Other Minor Disasters is funny, authentic, informative, and deeply compassionate. Dr. Menard encourages us all to learn from our mistakes and missteps and embrace our humanity as therapists. This is the book we all needed to read in graduate school to bring to life the human side of our profession. A must-read for every mental health professional whether newly accepted to their graduate program or therapists settled in their profession."

Dr. Tracy Dalgleish, author, psychologist, and couples therapist

Lessons from an Early Career Therapist

This book is a reassuring guide both for novice therapists and those further along in their journey, normalizing, validating, and empathizing with the human aspects of the profession and supporting readers to feel empowered and confident managing real-life situations with real-life clients.

Dr. Ménard shares lessons she learned in her early training years as well as those learned as a "grown-up" psychologist, addressing the perils and pitfalls of connecting with clients, working in diverse settings with different supervisors, balancing work and home life, and, perhaps most importantly, repairing and recovering from therapeutic stumbles and missteps with humor and compassion. Chapters address topics such as internship and licensure, therapist self-care, professionalism, diversity, supervision, and teletherapy and include important questions about clinical training and professional development like "What do I do when my client isn't making progress?", "How do I know when I'm too sick to work?", "Is it okay to curse in session?", "Do I even belong in this program?", and "What should I do if there is a wildlife invasion of my office?"

This book will provide mental health professionals with the tools and skills they need to problem-solve these situations and others on the road from graduate school and licensure to independent practice.

A. Dana Ménard, Ph.D., C.Psych, is an assistant professor of clinical psychology at the University of Windsor (Windsor, ON) and has held previous academic appointments at the University of Western Ontario (London, ON) and at Wayne State University (Detroit, MI). As a clinician, Dr. Ménard has worked at Detroit Receiving Hospital, the London Health Sciences Centre, the Royal Ottawa Hospital and the Ottawa Hospital, among others. She is the co-author of *Magnificent Sex: Lessons from Extraordinary Lovers* (2020, Routledge) with Dr. Peggy Kleinplatz, which won the 2021 Consumer Book Award from the Society of Sex Therapy and Research.

Lessons from an Early Career Therapist

Managing Mistakes, Missteps, and
Other Minor Disasters

A. Dana Ménard

Routledge
Taylor & Francis Group

NEW YORK AND LONDON

Designed cover image: Nicholas Armstrong

First published 2025
by Routledge
605 Third Avenue, New York, NY 10158

and by Routledge
4 Park Square, Milton Park, Abingdon, Oxon, OX14 4RN

Routledge is an imprint of the Taylor & Francis Group, an informa business

ISBN: 9781032409283 (hbk)
ISBN: 9781032409290 (pbk)
ISBN: 9781003355366 (ebk)

DOI: 10.4324/9781003355366

Typeset in Sabon
by Newgen Publishing UK

To John Trant,
for his love and support throughout this entire
journey

Contents

Acknowledgements

To my editor Julia Giordano and the rest of the staff at Routledge for helping me turn ideas into pages.

To Dr. Jessica Kichler, Dr. Alex Daros, Dr. Carlin Miller, and Dr. Aris Clemons, thank you for your thoughtful comments and suggestions. This book is much, much stronger because of the wisdom you shared so generously.

To my clients, thank you for your authenticity, for your commitment, for your humanity, and for the laughs. You were always my best teachers.

To my supervisees, thank you for your patience, for your enthusiasm, for challenging me, and for the fun we have learning together.

To my fellow students from graduate school and internship, thank you for the camaraderie in the trenches of higher education.

To all my clinical supervisors in graduate school, internship, and licensure. I am the psychologist I am now because of you, so really this is all your fault.

To my clinical colleagues of jobs past, thank you for your support and for your wisdom. Special thanks to Dr. Matt Ventimiglia for his advice during some of the trickier moments from Chapter 9.

To friends outside of clinical psychology, and in particular to Chelsea Honeyman, Alexis McBride, Michelle Bondy, John Hayward, and Claire Salisbury: thank you for the breaks, for the fun, for the support, for the perspective, and for the love.

To Dr. Margaret Echelbarger and the rest of the #100DaysofWriting crew: thank you for always being there when I needed some company and for endless cheerleading. I'm so glad I met you.

To my colleagues in the psychology department at the University of Windsor and especially the Council. Thank you for all the lessons I've begun to learn in the academic world!

To Connor Motzkus, for research help.

To Adam Libonati: thank you for loving Rosemary as though she were your own and for research assistance during her naps.

To my Dad, for his love and guidance throughout all these years. No thanks for his less-than-helpful advice during the possum episode. I miss you every day.

To Rosemary, thank you for being nothing more or less than the sunniest person I know. The world is better for having you in it.

To John, for his helpful commentary on early drafts and willingness to explain what joke he was laughing at, as well as general husbandly duties. Our journey together continues, and I look forward to doing it with you.

Introduction

I was 23 when I embarked on the educational journey that would one day lead to becoming a clinical psychologist. I was young and naïve – one might even say starry-eyed. I had grand visions about "rescuing" couples' marriages and helping clients to better understand their problems; most importantly, I wanted to *help* people. I was about to experience a very rude awakening. The next six years of graduate school were some of the most challenging and painful learning experiences I have ever had in my life, and that includes both (1) my semester of multivariate statistics and (2) a fencing class I took in undergrad. What followed was a lot of mistakes, missteps, and minor disasters, and a lot of lessons learned the hard way.

The training required to become a mental health professional is like no other type of training experience in life. No matter how many clinical books you read, how many session tapes you watch, how many friends you bully into letting you practice with them, nothing compares to the moment you and a client enter a therapy room for the first time and you actually try to help a real, live person; in that second, you go immediately from "not a therapist" to "a therapist." Don't worry, your clients can't hear you screaming on the inside (probably).

One major challenge associated with psychotherapy training requirements is the nature of the learning itself and how it relates to the personal qualities you possess as a human being. No other area of learning is likely to leave you feeling quite so vulnerable about the basic foundation of who you are as a person. For example, if you choose to study chemistry, you're learning about how to set up reactions and work safely with chemicals. If you study law, you're learning case history and how to speak in court. If you study communications...actually, I have no idea what those folks learn, but you probably get the gist of my argument. In most other programs, you are learning content and a set of skills for applying that content in the appropriate situations. In therapy training programs, you are

DOI: 10.4324/9781003355366-1

learning content, but the main set of skills you develop is how to create an effective, functional relationship with another person. The main "tool" of therapy, for lack of a better term, is you. So whereas a chemistry professor might say, "You didn't dilute that base properly," a clinical supervisor might say, "You weren't empathic enough when the client shared their trauma. You need to be warmer." That kind of feedback can be very tough to hear for beginning therapists because it can feel like a critique of your core personality.

Another factor that complicates this training is that the world of therapy contains very few clearly correct and clearly incorrect answers. Of course, there are some black-and-white issues, which we'll discuss later, but most of your other choices will be fairly subjective. Each session with each client will present dozens of branching possibilities; from one moment to the next, you'll need to decide what to do, what to say, how to say it, and when you should, in fact, say nothing at all. These choices are also likely to vary significantly from one setting to the next, one client to the next, and one supervisor to the next. Cognitive-behavioural techniques that you used routinely with one client may be less useful with another, who needs more interpersonal strategies. Swearing in session may be acceptable for some supervisors but would be verboten for others. Strategies that work in hospital settings may turn off private practice clients and vice versa. For me, graduate school required that I learn a different set of information and skills for working effectively in each setting every six months for about six years; not coincidentally, this was also the phase in my life when I finally began to drink coffee on a routine basis.

I think one of the main problems in how training programs prepare students to do clinical work is not that we don't recognize that the work itself is difficult, it's that we don't talk enough about the inevitability and, more importantly, acceptability of making mistakes. There was some discussion with my clinical supervisors around "do this" and "don't do this" but rather less discussion about what you should do if and when you got your wires crossed. Few of my clinical supervisors shared their mistakes, leading me to believe that they were perfect, infallible beings, emerging as fully formed psychologists from the brow of Freud, just as Athena sprung from the brow of Zeus. But learning how to translate mistakes into learning opportunities is an important piece of clinical growth and development and one of my main motivations for writing this book was to guide you in doing so yourself. My intent within these pages is to provide normalization, validation, and reassurance to you as you go through your own training process – you know, all that good stuff we tell clients to do for themselves but often forget to do for ourselves. I hope that this book will offer that to you through one of three routes:

(1) You will read this book, see the mistakes I've made, find empathy for similar mistakes you may have made, and feel better about who you are as a new clinician, or

(2) You will read this book, see the mistakes I've made, think to yourself, "Well, at least I never did *that*," and feel better about who you are as a new clinician, or

(3) You will read this book, see the mistakes I've made, and avoid them yourself (well done!).

Any approach you take is fine with me. Please think of this book as a buffet – feel free to pick and choose as you go along, taking double servings of what you need most and tiny scoops of ideas so outlandish they just might work.

What this book is

Before we go any further, let's be clear about what kind of lessons this book contains. I'm not here to talk about lessons learned from personal mistakes – those are just too embarrassing. I'm also not here to talk about research or teaching mistakes, although I've made a whole bunch of those too (for example, accidentally releasing a large swarm of angry bumblebees into the lab). We're here to talk about the many professional growth lessons I learned in graduate school and the first few years of independent practice as a clinical psychologist, and what you might take away from them for your own learning. During that time, I worked in a variety of different clinical settings and saw hundreds, if not thousands of clients from all walks of life.

Let's also be clear about who I am and where I'm coming from. I am a doctorate-level clinical psychologist specializing in adults and couples, so that's the training lens and the focus of the clinical experiences that I've had. Some you may be in counselling programs or nursing or social work or education or rehabilitation or something else entirely, and your program may therefore have varying degrees of similarity with mine. I'm hoping that these lessons may still be useful to you, even if your training and experiences are somewhat different. I must also be clear that the chapters in Part 2 (life as a "grown-up" psychologist) are specific to the settings and the populations with whom I've worked. I have certainly worked with a diverse group of patients at a variety of different settings including private practice, a trauma hospital, hospital outpatient clinics, and university counselling centres; however, I really can't speak to the challenges associated with certain kinds of presenting problems (e.g., eating disorders, alcohol/substance use) or that come from working with other populations such as children or families. I do expect some of these lessons may still translate; for example, when I told my friend who specializes in interventions with children and families that I was writing this book about lessons you don't learn in graduate school, she said, "Oh yeah, like that time a client took their shoe off and threw it at me!" I'm happy to report that I've never had to deal with projectiles in session. Another friend, who is a neuropsychologist, immediately brought up the time a client vomited on themselves in session; I am sad to report that my job has involved rather more bodily fluids than I would have expected based on what I was told in graduate school. So I am hopeful that some of this wisdom speaks to differences across settings, client groups, and training paradigms.

In summary, this book is a little bit about how to be a better therapist but it's mainly about how to be a happier, more relaxed therapist as you go through the learning and training process. It's intended to help you sit in the therapist chair with more comfort and more confidence, no matter whether it's a comfy armchair in private practice or one of those hard plastic numbers that hospitals use exclusively for their group therapy rooms.

Chapter roadmap

Part 1 of the book is intended to cover lessons that may be particularly relevant during your graduate education and early practical work experiences. Chapters 1 and 2 will cover lessons specific to the process of clinical training. For me, the initial learning curve was nearly vertical and there were a lot of crucial lessons I wish I had figured out sooner like "Are all the other trainees better than me?" and "How can I make myself a better therapist faster?" We'll cover important concepts like whether you should swear an undying allegiance to one therapeutic orientation, who is most responsible for change during the psychotherapy process (hint: it's not you), and whether the children's show *Bluey* should be required viewing for aspiring psychotherapists. Chapter 3 will address lessons learned in clinical supervision such as how and when to speak up about your needs and concerns and whether you ever get used to the sound of your own voice on therapy recordings. Chapter 4 covers issues related to the internship and licensure years, including how often to tabulate your clinical hours, how to manage application stress, and how to cope when you realize that you've become the adultiest adult in the room. Chapter 5 addresses lessons related to self-care and mental health. Taking care of yourself so that you can take care of others is a crucial lesson for most clinicians, but many of us struggle with walking the walk, even when we talk the talk all day long. Chapter 6 focuses on the sometimes controversial and often nebulous concept of "professionalism." We'll tackle challenging topics like social media use, hugging your clients, and whether it's okay to drink water in session.

Part 2 focuses on lessons I learned as a post-graduate in the "real world" of clinical practice. Chapter 7 cover lessons from work I did in outpatient settings including psychiatric hospitals, student counselling centres, and private practice. We'll tackle questions like, "How can I help someone when their insurance only covers three sessions?" and "Should you shell out $1,500 for that airport hotel workshop?" Chapter 8 is focused specifically on working with couples and will address my early misconception about whether or not you can "rescue" marriages. Chapter 9 addresses issues that arose from working in inpatient settings from the highly conceptual – "How do you creatively adapt evidence-based strategies to apply in situations where a patient's autonomy may be limited?" – to the very basic – "How do you cope with bad smells on the job?" Chapter 10 will address challenges related to working with a diverse clientele because I feel confident that what the world of psychotherapy really needs to address complex, long-standing issues faced by minoritized and marginalized people is another white woman's opinion (just kidding). Chapter 11 will focus on lessons learned as a supervisor and how I managed when the shoe was finally on the other foot. Chapter 12 is about virtual therapy and covers how what I learned from researching great sex (Kleinplatz & Ménard, 2020) applies to the world of psychotherapy (hint: it involves Vaseline).

I have included examples throughout the book of interactions I've had with various clients but in these cases, potentially identifying information like gender, age, ethnicity, etc. has been changed. If you think you recognize your annoying cousin Diane in these pages because I talk about doing therapy with a young, Asian woman with relationship troubles, it's far more likely that the real client was an older gay Black man.

Part 1

The training years

Chapter 1

Junior grad student

Greetings

Congratulations! After many years of hard work, you've finally been accepted by your dream graduate program. You're about to embark on the journey that will eventually lead to you being a licensed therapist. In just a few short years, you'll have your own clients, your own office, your own therapy couch, and your very own closet full of cardigans – I'm sorry but this part of the uniform is mandatory.

That was the good news. This is the bad news: learning how to be a mental health professional may be the hardest thing you've ever learned how to do in your whole life. Harder than learning to drive, harder than high school gym class, harder even than getting over the last season of *Game of Thrones*. If you completed your undergraduate degree through that trusted cycle of memorizing content, regurgitating it for tests, and then forgetting it, this learning process is likely to be a rude awakening. You can't read your way into being a good therapist and there's nothing to memorize. Rather, it's about learning how to create a relationship with another human that's utterly different from any other kind of relationship you've had in your life, and the learning curve on how to make that happen is really, really steep.

Let me assure you, you will survive. It is very likely, if not inevitable, that you will feel overwhelmed from time-to-time, and you may wonder if you've picked the right path and whether you'll ever get through your degree. I can say with almost complete certainty that you did and you will, especially if you have the right attitude – and you bought this book, so I think you do! Dozens of people have survived these training programs and gone on to become flourishing clinicians and amazing role models for their colleagues and clients. And the rest of us are getting by as well as we can.

Now that I've scared the crap out of you, let's spend the rest of the chapter talking about how to manage that anxiety, shall we? Trust me, if

DOI: 10.4324/9781003355366-3

we work together, we can take your emotions down from a 9/10 to a solid 6/10 (where 10 is the most anxious you've ever felt in your life and 0 is a monk on Ativan). Also, please get used to rating emotions on a 10-point scale, you're going to be doing it a lot.

A word of caution before we begin: you may find yourself rolling your eyes here and there, especially in these first couple of chapters. This stuff may seem terribly obvious, barely worth mentioning let alone including in a book. "What kind of therapist," you ask yourself, "would forget that the client is the main determinant of therapy success?" Well, me, for one. I've done this repeatedly. Most of the graduate students I've supervised. Probably you too, at some point. I think ideas become cliché because they are the types of thoughts that are so fundamental, so basic and so obvious, so embarrassingly simple that they're easy to overlook. See also me forgetting to introduce myself to my clients at their initial intake (more on that later this chapter). It's hard to believe that such simple ideas could be so important and when they're brought to your attention, you feel a bit silly, but I think it's human nature to over-focus on complexity and overlook the fundamentals, at least from time to time. It's easy to fixate on fancy techniques or the newest three-letter acronym therapy and forget the basics, but those basics are often crucial to success, both with clients and in getting yourself through your training in one piece.

You already have a lot going for you

If you are the kind of person who wants to be a therapist, you've probably got a good foundation for this work personality-wise: you care about other people, you want to help them with their troubles, you listen well, you're empathic and probably a bunch of other warm-and-fuzzy qualities too (Hill et al., 2013). Maybe you just have the kind of face that makes people on public transportation start telling you about their troubles; this is called "Resting Talk-to-me Face" and we'll address it later (see Chapter 6, p. 5). These qualities matter and are relevant, so try to remember this when you're feeling overwhelmed and daunted by your training.

Years ago, I told a supervisor that I didn't want to matter to my clients. My deeply flawed logic was that if I became too important to them, my mistakes would have a correspondingly greater ability to wound or hurt them, and I didn't want to let anyone down or disappoint them. She patiently listened to this nonsense and then said something very useful: the kinds of mistakes you make when something is important to you and you're trying very hard to be good at it are different from the kinds of mistakes you make when you just don't care about something and are being thoughtless. This is an excellent point. For example, you will definitely, at some point in your training, misunderstand something the client has said to you or forget some details about their lives; this is normal and happens even to the most experienced therapists. However, if you care about being a good therapist, it is unlikely that you will miss it because you were deliberately ignoring them during the session or surreptitiously looking at your phone. If you are putting in lots of effort to become a better therapist and looking for opportunities to learn and grow and develop, you will still make mistakes, but they'll be different from the kinds of mistakes you'd make if you didn't want to be here at all and you couldn't care less about the kind of therapist you will become.

Find a way to remind yourself of this. You have some important, fundamental qualities that will stand you in good stead throughout your training program and your career. And if you sometimes struggle to find the energy to remind yourself, remind your classmates because they could probably do with the refresher themselves.

You won't be able to do it all

Most training programs in the helping professions require a very competitive entry process. You need high grades, stellar extracurriculars, research experience, glowing letters of reference, straight teeth, a resting heart rate of 50, the ability to speak to birds...you know, normal human stuff. You would hope, perhaps, that after having fought your way into the program that the road ahead would be smooth and pleasant after the battle to get there. Sadly, this is unlikely to be the case. Now you're going to be asked to balance a full courseload, clinical training, research, and teaching assistanceships, and possibly also, depending on your career goals, applying for scholarships, writing up journal articles, attending conferences or workshops, sitting comprehensive examinations, and applying for competitive internships. Here's the really tricky adjustment: the mindset that got you into this program is now your worst enemy. You may believe that "A"s got you here so "A"s will be crucial to getting through this next phase of your training as well. Your brain is likely to continue to insist on "A" effort across the spectrum of your activities: "A"s in courses, "A"s in clinical training, "A"s in research, "A"s in marking undergraduates' midterm exams. This is a very unhelpful mentality and likely to cause significant stress. Or, to put it another way, your brain can be a real "A"-hole in graduate school.

Simply put, this is not feasible: you will burn out, you will start to hate your classes, your research, your supervisors, your colleagues, and your clients, not to mention your past self for having the dumb idea to pursue this career in the first place. Research has established that self-critical perfectionism – the idea that you're never good enough and aren't living up to your own high standards – is highly related to higher depression and burnout (Richardson et al., 2020). I urge you not to let yourself get to this point. Instead, embrace a shift to a "good enough" mentality. Did you get enough of your readings done that you can hold your own in a class discussion? Good enough! Did you get a messy first draft of your ethics application submitted to your supervisor? Good enough! Did you get your session notes written up by overusing three verbs? Good enough! Did you give up half-way through marking the undergraduates' midterms and just use the "staircase method", i.e., throw them down the stairs and the exams at the top get the highest marks, those at the bottom get the lowest? Uh, no, don't do that last one.

You do need to get everything done but that last 10–20% of work in each category is probably not going to make the difference between "winning an award for clinical excellence" and "the worst therapist who ever lived." Did you ever hear that old joke about what you call the medical student at the bottom of the class?[1] You need to learn to ignore your little perfectionist voice: decide what "good enough" looks like for a particular task, put in the necessary amount of work to get there, and then just walk away. See Chapter 5 on self-care for activities you could be doing instead with this found time.

Run the mile you're in

I took up long-distance running while I was in graduate school because the only thing smarter than being in a masochistic academic program is having a masochistic hobby to fill the off hours. There's a proverb in the running community that is often applied to long-distances races: run the mile you're in (Canadian runners are free to substitute "kilometer" as preferred). The idea is that if you're doing a road race and you keep focusing on just how long that race is and how much total time you're going to be running, there's a real danger that you'll get overwhelmed and, soon after, demoralized. At best, the running will seem a lot harder and less enjoyable; at worst, you might just talk yourself into quitting despite all the hard work you put in to getting there. Here is an example of *not* running the mile you're in: a couple of years into my Ph.D., I sat down and calculated how many days I had remaining in the degree – over 800 days, at that point. As you might have predicted, this information did not help to motivate me in the slightest or, as a friend in the same program put it, "What were you *trying* to accomplish?"

Run the mile you're in: true for long-distance races and true for psychotherapy training programs. Don't think about running the whole

---

1 Doctor! Yuk, yuk.

marathon (26.2 miles – eep!), think about the mile that you are currently running. Don't think about all your training requirements – the classes, the clinical hours, the research, the internship, the licensing. Ask yourself instead: what's the next thing I have to do? Get through your courses this semester? Get a section of your thesis proposal done? Research clinical settings for your next placement? If those steps seem too big for you, break them into even smaller chunks. What is the smallest step you can take that will move you forward, maintain your momentum, and build your self-confidence? Is it sending an email to your committee? Is it opening up your email, typing your committee members' addresses into the "to" line and then calling it a day? Forward motion is still forward motion, even if it's small, slow, or incomplete.

The small steps approach is helpful for all aspects of your training as it's very easy to get lost at times with how much new information you're learning and how many new skills you're trying to develop. Consider picking just one thing every week and focus on running that particular mile. Maybe you want to develop your capacity for sitting in silence during the session. So just do that: for every client and every session that week, look for your chance to use silence more effectively, or you might decide that your one goal this week is to write your notes as efficiently as possible, or it might be to tune in and notice what's happening in your body when the client is speaking, or it might be to ask better open-ended questions. Just pick something, spend some time on it, and then pick the next thing. Over time, you will cover the full distance with your small, forward steps.

Side note: I ran my first full marathon in 2017 while I was working a hospital job and spending about half my working hours supervising the clinical work of graduate students. One of my students was also a long-distance runner, albeit a much, much faster one. When I limped into work on the Monday after the race and told him that I had successfully completed the whole 26.2 miles, he asked me if my finishing time should best be measured in hours or days. For more on how to respond to that kind of back-talk from trainees, see Chapter 11.

Your clients are more afraid of you than you are of them

In the first year of seeing actual, real clients, I had an upset stomach before most of my sessions. I tried to manage this by repeating "you're fine, you're fine, you're fine" over and over again in my head, but my stomach just wasn't buying it. There were many contributors to this anxiety. I was worried that I would miss something important, forget to ask about important details or blank on how to do an intervention properly. Mainly, I was worried that I would not be "A Good Therapist," whatever that means. When reviewing the videotapes of my sessions, I would catch myself nervously picking at my fingernails and fidgeting, but you know what I didn't see on the tapes? My clients noticing my anxiety and then loudly and belligerently expressing their doubts about my ability to help them with their problems. Instead, they behaved like people with troubles who believed that I was there to help and do my best, which was true despite all the nerves and stomach distress.

Many clients wait months or even years to go to therapy (Vogel et al., 2007). They may be psyching themselves up to share an issue or a secret that they have literally never shared with another human being. They may be terrified of being judged or shamed; they may be feeling hopeless about their current situation or paralyzed with unhappiness. "Am I the craziest person you've ever met?" is a question I've gotten on a monthly basis throughout my career. They may have all kinds of stigmatizing beliefs in their heads about what it means to have mental health issues or to be in therapy (Clement et al., 2015). In short: clients have a lot going on. They're generally too preoccupied with their own stuff to worry about you much beyond "Are they a genuine person who's doing their best to listen to my problems and help me?" The number of clients who have outwardly expressed doubt about my abilities to help is very low, and usually more a reflection on their interpersonal style than a real concern.

I'm not saying you shouldn't worry at all about being a good therapist – you can and should be concerned about what kind of practitioner you are – but the standard to which you hold yourself is likely to be far, far higher than your clients' standards for you. In those first few sessions, they're far more likely to be focused on their own pain and stress that brought them into therapy than on you. If you are warm, empathic, non-judgmental, and listen to them, your relationship will be off to a great start.

Avoid orientation dogmatism

About three months into my clinical psychology Ph.D., I was asked to identify my therapeutic orientation during a classroom exercise. The idea even then struck me as absurd – I hadn't even sat in a room with a client yet! Isn't that what I was here to find out? How could I answer such an important question based on a few undergraduate classes? However, no one else in the class said "I don't know yet" so I said something about Rogers and humanism, the professor [a Cognitive Behavioural Therapy (CBT) devotee] gave me a funny look, and we moved on. Except I clearly haven't because I'm now writing about this incident 15 years later.

To me, being asked to swear allegiance to one approach with all clients forever and ever is absurd, like choosing one type of food to serve at all meals with all guests under all circumstances. Can you imagine having chili for breakfast, lunch, and dinner every day? Sometimes you need a nice, crunchy salad instead. Sometimes I want to order Chinese food, but my dining companion had a bad experience with Chinese food last week and wants something different. Sometimes people have allergies and intolerances, so you do your usual curry recipe but leave out the coconut milk or the cilantro.

Research has repeatedly shown that most practicing psychotherapists identify as integrative or eclectic in their orientation (Goodyear et al., 2016; Heinonen & Orlinsky, 2013), and I don't think that's an accident. It seems like most of us prefer the buffet approach: traditional desensitization techniques for a spider phobia, interpersonal strategies for conflict with mom. Even the illustrious founders of psychotherapy were known to stray from the commandments they laid down. For example, in his excellent book *The Gift of Therapy*, Yalom describes how Freud strayed from the "blank-screen" model he advocated for psychoanalysis (2017, p. 76). If Freud himself didn't strictly follow the rules he laid down for operating within the framework of one particular therapeutic orientation, I don't think the rest of us need to either.

As a practicing psychologist, I've rarely had clients ask me for many details about my approach to therapy. Now and then, a client will specifically ask for CBT but usually when questioned further, they don't know themselves what the acronym stands for or what it involves. Rather, the usual response is some version of "My doctor said I needed CBT," likely because this was the only approach to therapy covered during the physician's time in medical school. Other clients don't know that there are different schools of thought on how to bring about therapeutic change and will look incredulous when you tell them that thousands of people have collectively spent millions of hours arguing with one another about which one is better.

It's definitely worthwhile to pick an approach or two and understand them in greater depth so that you can give this framework to clients and help them make sense of their issues. Research supports the idea that clients improve when they can understand and explain the connections between their symptoms and their problems (Crits-Christoph et al., 2003; Jennissen et al., 2018). If a specific model makes good sense to you, you'll be able to explain it well and if you can explain it well, clients will understand it well and will then be able to use it themselves. But don't feel you need to pick something in your first class and then stick with it forever and ever, with no deviations. Unless you like having chili at every meal, in which case more power to you.

Be yourself in therapy

At some point during your training, you may find yourself tempted to try to imitate another clinician that you feel is very effective and does really good work with their clients. Your mind may tell you that you too could have similarly amazing results if you changed your tone of voice, if you added better non-verbal responses, if you could just perfect your "empathetic listening" face (hint: it's all in the eyebrow movement).

In my case, it was someone else who was telling me to imitate another person's approach. The professor supervising my very first clinical case felt that I wasn't speaking slowly or softly enough to amplify the emotions my client was experiencing in session. I wasn't doing enough non-verbal follows and my "Mmmhmm"s were terrible. The supervisor encouraged me to model my approach after my colleague Ashley, who was also in our supervision group, and who was getting better results with her non-verbals than I was. Rather than just be angry at Ashley for wrecking the grading curve for the rest of us, I resolved to do better. I walked into my next session with a mission and spent the therapeutic hour patiently waiting for an opportunity to demonstrate my prowess at these skills. Finally, it happened! The client shared a recent emotional experience and I responded with my very best, most prolonged, most heartfelt and emotion-inducing "Mmmmmm, mmmmhmmm", complete with sympathetic head tilt and nod. It took a good five seconds to get it out. My client paused to observe this travesty of acting and burst out laughing – uncontrollable, tear-streaming belly laughing. I was mortified, and for a few seconds, I completely froze. Nothing in my training had prepared me for how to respond when your client starts laughing at you. And then I started laughing too. The client was right: it was so over the top and put-on and inauthentic. Frankly, I'm just grateful that the client laughed instead of saying "What the hell was that?"

During your training, you will encounter supervisors who will push you to try different approaches and styles and you should give these things a try, but you must also stay grounded in who you are. Deepen and expand your natural expressions of empathy, of curiosity, of cheerleading, but don't try to adopt wholesale someone else's approach. I learned a very important lesson that day: there are many right ways to be a warm, empathetic therapist but most of them will probably involve some version of your natural speaking voice.

You are not the main contributor to your client's improvement

You are about to spend the next few years of your life learning everything you can about assessment and intervention. You're going to learn theories of change, developmental models, and all the different ways those can go wrong. You'll learn techniques and worksheets and therapeutic exercises – oh my! As you desperately try to stuff all of this information into your brain, make sure you don't forget the person who is most in control of the client's improvement: the client themselves. This is the number one factor that predicts whether or not therapy is successful. Study after study shows that the biggest predictors of change are (1) client factors (Bohart & Tallman, 2010; Greenberg et al., 2006) and (2) the therapeutic alliance (Baier et al., 2020; Norcross & Lambert, 2018). You have no control over item #1 and only partial control over item #2. Specific therapeutic techniques account for only about 15% of improvement in therapy (Cooper, 2008) so if you ever find yourself laying awake at night thinking, "If only I knew how to do a proper two-chair technique, they'd get better," give yourself a shake. This is very, very unlikely.

I need you to internalize this lesson so let's do a little thought experiment with a different field: if someone took piano lessons but never practiced, would they learn how to play? Would it matter if the teacher was really, really good and knew all the latest techniques and piano-teaching philosophies? What if the teacher lay awake at night dreaming up ways to be a better teacher and somehow get through to this student? What if they read 18 books on how to be a better piano teacher and role-played new strategies with all their piano-teaching colleagues? Would any of this matter to a student who had no interest in learning piano whatsoever and who was only there because mom said they couldn't play video games unless they attended their lessons? I'd be willing to bet a lot of money that the student in these scenarios is learning very little music. Trust me, this is a perfect analogy: I've had some parents threaten to take away their teenager's video games unless they came to therapy, and it produces the exact level of motivation for active participation in therapy that you're probably picturing (zero).

Clients come to therapy at all different stages of readiness. Sometimes they are ready to move and make changes on some issues but not on others. Sometimes, they seem hardly prepared to move on any issue. Sometimes, clients will have a very clear goal in mind and work as hard as they can, but they still won't have completely achieved it by the end of therapy. All of these scenarios are okay and none of them mean that therapy has failed. Sometimes, the work of therapy is planting seeds that will only come to fruition later. The difficult part for you, the therapist, is that you won't know which of the above situations applies to your case until quite a way along. In one case, I had been seeing a client for over a year for anxiety and depression. We explored the idea that the boredom and frustration they were experiencing at work was probably feeding their depression and that they might be better working in the field for which they had trained. When we wrapped up therapy, they were still working their frustrating position and their progress in several areas had been limited by that. However, years later, I saw a newspaper article featuring a large photo of my client with a write-up about the successful business they had started in their field.

They looked so happy that if I hadn't seen their name in print, I wouldn't have recognized them.

Turn it into your own personal mantra and repeat it often: the client is in charge of their own change process. Write it in your journal, maybe embroider it on a pillow if you're the crafty type, but find a way to remember it.

Don't let other clinicians "psych" you out

Early on in my training, I remember sitting in a class that included several students further along than I was – naturally, I saw these students as role models, the "big kids" of the psychology graduate program. They so obviously had their stuff together: their outfits were coordinated, their hairstyles were on point, they never seemed to be carrying too many bags. One of them used to carry around an actual china teacup on an actual china saucer from class to class – this was clearly someone who had her life well-organized.

On that particular day, one of these senior students airily volunteered that earlier in her practice, she used to focus on the content of what clients were saying but had now switched almost exclusively to commenting on the therapeutic process. The exact details of the client's experience, she implied, were comparatively unimportant. "Goodness!" I thought to myself. "This person who has her stuff together doesn't worry about the content of the session. Maybe I, too, should focus much harder on the process and ignore the details?" In the weeks that followed, I did my best to spend more time at the process level, feeling like an immature novice when I found myself caught up in details and content.

There is a lot of wisdom to the idea of attending to process, but let me tell you a different story from much later in my career. I was a "grown-up" psychologist who had been fully licensed for several years and I was working with a student who was struggling to complete a class. We spent a lot of time addressing the roots of their procrastination and their fears and doubts about their academic program, but the student continued to struggle. They were finding it impossible to complete their final assignment for the course and had blown not only the original deadline, but several extensions negotiated with the professor. After weeks of escalating conflict that eventually included my client, their professor, the teaching assistant for the course, a student experience officer, and a lesser vice president in their faculty, I thought to ask the student what the assignment was worth. "5%" they replied, meaning that the student was going to pass the course with or without this assignment. I couldn't believe that I'd overlooked something so relevant to the problem. This was an extremely important detail and likely would have changed my whole approach to the situation.

So what have we learned? Process is definitely important but under no circumstances should you ignore the details of a client's situation lest they come back to bite you both. And what else have we learned? No matter how well-dressed someone is, or how confidently they speak, or even whether they carry china teacups around, there's no one right answer to doing good therapy. There is no one approach, no way of being, no orientation or exercise that's just the best way to do therapy, so don't let anyone tell you otherwise.

Practice your words

Have you ever watched a competitive baking show, like *The Great British Baking Show* or its Canadian equivalent (fundamentally the same, just with more maple syrup)? I love these shows so much, but they're so deceptive. In any given week, some accountant named Joe will make the perfect apple tart and you'll think to yourself, "I could do that!" You then try it yourself and accidentally leave out the apples. The difference is that Joe has made a hundred apple tarts and he's already made all the mistakes one could make in the baking of apple tarts; the effortlessness you see on screen is all part of his hard-won tart-making skill.

Learning to talk to real-life clients is very similar. The therapy training videos, the dialogues in textbooks, and the demonstrations from your professors are deceptive: these people have been doing this work for years and they are fluent in "wording things appropriately for clients." For them, it is largely effortless because they've said variations on these themes a hundred times, so it requires a lot less brainpower. But you, my friend, are going to need to think quite hard about your wording, at least initially. You may be surprised to find how big a difference there can be between knowing something in your head versus expressing it fluently. In your initial sessions, the situation is likely to be compounded by the nerves you're feeling because eeks, this is a real-life client who actually expects me to help them and not Becky from my class who's just playing a client and keeps giggling!

You need to practice your words. Find willing friends and family members – grudgingly willing is fine – and practice introducing yourself, explaining the structure of therapy and sessions, going through the limits of confidentiality, providing the instructions for a worksheet or in-session exercise. Practice anything that you might eventually have to say to a real-life client. This is the time for you to trip over your sentences, leave out something important, or get a detail wrong. Achieving fluid therapy verbiage is like any other skill, it gets better with practice; over time, you'll try different wordings with different clients and you'll naturally figure out how to express yourself. But in the meantime, practice so that when you leave the metaphorical apples out of your metaphorical therapy tart, it's with a classmate instead of a real-life client.

Make your peace with mistakes

As an early-career clinician, you are about to make a lot of mistakes, and what's more, you will continue making mistakes long past the time you might have hoped they would stop. Allow me to illustrate with a personal example that happened several years after I had graduated with a Ph.D. I was working in private practice and I brought a new couple in from the waiting room to get started on the usual new client activities: filling in paperwork, going through the limits of confidentiality, and discussing the intake process. At the end of this, I asked if they had any questions. "Yes," said the husband, "Is the psychologist coming or...?" I had forgotten to introduce myself and he was unsure whether I was their actual provider or merely the paperwork gal. We had a good laugh and then had a good first session.

At one point in my career, I hoped that I would someday get to a point where there would be no more mistakes; I now know that that magical day will likely be the one right before I hang up my therapist cardigan or, more likely, never. But that's okay because a lot of mistakes aren't serious mistakes, and a lot of them may be fixable. What's more, the process of fixing your mistakes may actually be a valuable experience for the client. If you didn't spend enough time on something that is important to the client, it is more than likely that the issue will come up again until you correctly identify it. If you said something that the client found invalidating, hopefully, they'll react and/or bring it up and you can explore that experience. If you double-book clients or start a session late because you got distracted, you can apologize, take responsibility, and try to make it right. For some of your clients, this will be the first time that anyone in their lives has been so respectful and taken responsibility for their screw-up. It can be a valuable therapeutic intervention for you to demonstrate (1) that even good people can make mistakes, (2) that mistakes can be put right, and (3) and we can all move on.

Start a diary

This is one piece of advice that I will freely admit I didn't take, mostly because no one told me to, but I really wish I had, and not just because it would have made writing this book way easier. It can be very, very hard to track the development of your clinical skills. There's no exam you can take, no pop-up that will let you know that your empathy is up 17% over this time last year. It's hard to know for certain that you now have more confidence working with a certain kind of client or with a certain kind of problem than you did when you first started. Part of the problem is that if you keep pushing yourself, you'll always feel on the edge of discomfort because there's always more to know and learn. But unlike lifting dumb-bells, where you can see that you've moved from the 5 lb weights to the 15 lb weights, it's harder to compare your progress as a clinician. The only way you will know is if you have a way to check in with your past self.

Consider keeping a record of some kind and checking in regularly so that you can see how you're growing as a clinician. It could be a paper journal or a digital diary or a running note on your phone but find a way to track your progress. Ask yourself what's going really well these days? Where do you feel you've made improvements? What's challenging you right this minute? Where do you want to be in a week, a month, or a year? What problems or populations do you want to gain experience with and what have you learned from the experiences you've had? If you don't know where to start, how about this: on the first page, write down your reasons for going into the field. The next few years may be rough, and it will be good to have a visual reminder of why you're putting yourself through this when your mind will be begging you to consider literally any other career option (for example, dog walker, bakery owner, crime-fighting librarian). Down the road, when you're struggling or feeling demoralized, re-read the journal and see how far you've come in your knowledge and skills. That way, you can remember that time you forgot to introduce yourself to a client and feel better about the mistakes you've fixed.

Conclusion

Becoming a therapist is a lifelong learning process and you can't rush it. You certainly can't accelerate your progress at the beginning, when you're probably at your most anxious and would desperately like to do so. You can't read yourself into being a better therapist. I know: I tried. Learning the ropes of therapy will require thousands of hours of practice, super-vision, reading, watching tapes, and taking classes and workshops. The learning is so gradual, so imperceptible that sometimes you won't even realize that it's happening. Rest assured that it is and be patient with your-self. You deserve to be here.

Chapter 2

Senior grad student

Learning to be a therapist is a lot like learning to drive: initially, you need complete silence from everyone else in the vehicle so that you can focus, grip the steering wheel so hard your fingers turn white, and whip your head around like a nervous parrot. Over time, hopefully, you will begin to relax and become more confident in the basic skills, at which point you can turn your attention to more complex problems like learning how to drive a stick shift or on a major highway during rush hour. Therapy is very similar: once you've mastered the basics, you can take on some bigger challenges and sharpen your skills. Here are some of the lessons I learned after I got over (some of) the initial terror.

Clients don't know "the rules"

After you've been "therapisting" for a while, the rules of therapy may start to become second-nature to you. You know, for example, that there are limits to confidentiality, that physical touching of clients is generally off-limits, and that you can't give someone a lift home after the session. However, you must always keep in mind that clients don't know these rules, as many of them have never done any kind of therapy. Some of them have been exposed through friends and family who have done it, but a size-able portion are likely to have learned everything they know about therapy from movies, television, and books (McDonald et al., 2014). This is a major issue for a couple of reasons. For a start, television and movie plots almost always revolve around therapists behaving unethically (Wahl et al., 2018), often in flagrant, horrifying ways. Thankfully, this has not been a significant issue with most of my clients: they generally know without being told that I'm not going to be their date to a family member's wedding or take them on some kind of whirlwind "manic pixie dream girl" type adventure to show them their true priorities in life. However, in addition to these misrepresentations, television and movies almost never depict the less-interesting bits like completing forms at the start of an intake session.

DOI: 10.4324/9781003355366-4

For example, I could never really get into *The Sopranos* because the first session between Tony and his therapist *doesn't* start with her explaining the limits of confidentiality. I've been told by fans of the show that the ethical violations didn't stop there; possibly these could have been avoided had she started by communicating appropriate boundaries.

A few years ago, I had a new client on my schedule at a university counselling centre. My office was in an odd spot and could be quite difficult to locate so I asked them, "Did you have any trouble finding my office?" I thought it was a nice, neutral opening question. Here's the dialogue that ensued.

Client: Oh yeah, my buddy Brad showed me. You're seeing him for therapy too.
Me: Oh, um. [pause] I really can't say anything about that.
Client: No, he said it's cool. He walked me to your office.
Me: Uh, I *really* can't say anything about my other clients. [desperately]
Client: He said you were super-helpful.
Me: Uh....let's fill out these three forms.

This situation made perfect sense to both clients: the first client liked me, so he recommended me to his friend. In the outside world, this kind of behaviour is natural. You see a hair stylist you like, you recommend them to a friend and maybe you both get a discount but in the therapy world, you can't talk about who else you're seeing, and there aren't usually discounts.

Once you've explained the limits of confidentiality a few hundred times or the standard protocols for psychotherapy at your work site, it will be easy to go into "robot mode" with your clients and rush through explanations at lightning speed. Try not to. Even as the rules become fully automatic and obvious to you, they won't be to your clients. You have to imagine that every client has no idea how therapy goes and that you will be guiding them through every step to make sure you both stay on the same page. Assume that any new client may know nothing at all about the process and content of psychotherapy and that you will be both doing the work with them and simultaneously explaining what the work is and why you're doing it. And don't be surprised if clients recommend you to their friends, just don't confirm (or deny!) that you're seeing those friends.

Client self-awareness

Clients can be surprisingly self-aware about some very dysfunctional behaviours in their life, but them demonstrating this level of insight in their discussions with you doesn't always mean that they're ready, willing, or able to do anything about it. In other words, people can have a very good understanding of their own bullshit but still be completed trapped by it. (See also me standing in the cookie aisle at the grocery store rationalizing to myself that this time, I will certainly eat only the recommended serving of Oreos and *not* half a package in one sitting.) No matter your preferred psychotherapeutic orientation, I think all clinicians can benefit from reading about Prochaska and DiClemente's transtheoretical model of change (1983); spend some extra time on the "contemplation" stage to understand the thought processes of clients who have some level of insight but who are not yet ready to make big changes.

In one of my early placements in graduate school, I worked at a clinic that offered support for smoking cessation. A client came in for an initial session but said that they were still feeling very uncertain about quitting smoking and were unsure when and how they wanted to move forward. I said that was fine and we made an appointment to further explore this ambivalence and consider the pros and cons of quitting smoking. The client cancelled their follow-up. No problem, we rescheduled. They cancelled that appointment too. We rescheduled again. They didn't show up to the next appointment and didn't call. All told, the client cancelled or no-showed to five separate sessions before me, my supervisor, and the client all collectively threw in the towel. This was beyond aggravating to me as a student trying to get my clinical training done, but I couldn't fault the client: they had told me exactly what they were thinking at the very first session. However, merely having this insight about uncertainty and ambivalence didn't provide enough motivation for them to lean into those feelings and really explore them.

Sometimes, it may feel that developing client insight and self-awareness is half the battle in therapy, if not more. If they're already aware of their problematic patterns, you might think, they're that much further ahead and it won't be long before the client breaks free. And they might be! You might be lucky enough to be the therapist in the room when everything clicks, and the client is finally able to move on from a long-standing issue. But don't take it personally or see it as a reflection on your therapy skills if that doesn't happen over the current course of therapy. Sometimes we're just a drop of water among many others slowly wearing away the rock below; it's going to take many more drops before anything really changes. Both roles are valuable.

"I thought about that thing you said" (client version)

I've heard these words so many times from clients in therapy, and they always produce a sense of disquiet in me as soon as I hear them because it's almost never a carefully thought-out insight or a beautiful therapeutic metaphor or even a deeply empathic statement about the client's current emotional state. More often than not, it's some off-the-cuff BS that I casually tossed out without a second thought and that may or may not be grounded in scientific research or the therapy literature. Now, sometimes it's incredibly useful BS that the client has been waiting to hear and that was the key to unlocking a deeper understanding of their issues but I still feel vaguely ashamed every time.

It's impossible for us to know which comments are really going to resonate with clients (Bachelor, 2013; Chui et al., 2020). It's also impossible, as far as I know, for human therapists to sound deeply therapist-y with every remark they make in a session. Invariably, some casual remark or flippant response is going to resonate with the client even if that was not our intention. Embrace it. I say this partly because you really don't have a choice, but also because these types of remarks can be extremely helpful. My theory is that clients know that these comments are authentic, and maybe that's why they stick so well. I recommend that you follow up to find out why that comment in particular was so useful and why it stuck out among the sea of other deeply incisive and thoughtful comments with which I'm sure you filled the therapy hour.

I think these moments also remind us to be humble as therapists. Dr. Irvin D. Yalom, an expert in both existential psychotherapy and group approaches, once co-wrote an entire book about the course of psychotherapy alongside a client who was an aspiring writer, with each chapter alternating between his reflections on a therapy session and then hers (Yalom & Elkin, 1991). In some instances, they both had entirely different perspectives on the same therapy hour and entirely different takeaways. What we expect the client to get from therapy and what they actually get from it may often be different, but that doesn't mean either party is wrong, it's just a question of perspective and what each person needs from that hour.

Sometimes when a client makes reference to something you supposedly said in a previous session, it's followed by a comment that you *definitely* did not make. It may even be a piece of advice or a clinical recommendation that is not at all consistent with your treatment plan, or even with good clinical practice, but rather something that the client just really wanted to hear. For example, that it would be just fine to continue avoiding their anxiety triggers or that yelling at a coworker is the ideal way to resolve interpersonal conflict in the workplace. In this case, don't be surprised if the client clings to their version of what they wished you'd said despite your gentle corrections. It can be annoying to have bad advice attributed to you but it's a valuable insight into the client's thought processes.

Whether the client is accurate or not and whether they cite a profound thought you shared or just a side comment, it's valuable information to know what they are taking away from a therapy session. In a similar vein,

I can only assume that your main takeaway from this book will not be some beautifully worded and carefully cited paragraph of clinical wisdom but rather a stupid joke or story that makes me look foolish (the possum story from Chapter 6 comes to mind). And I'm (mostly) okay with that.

Don't fall for branding

As you progress through your training, you may have the opportunity to attend workshops or training programs to learn about therapeutic approaches. ACT, CBT, EFT, DBT, IFS[1] – more than likely it will be an approach referred to by a three-letter acronym because that's how we like it in the world of psychotherapy. It's worth going to a few here and there, if you have the time and money; however, when you're picking and choosing, try to focus on the basics of established approaches, and most importantly, watch out for marketing hype. Therapy is like any other area of human interest: it goes through trends, some of which are benign and some of which are decidedly less so (Paris, 2023). It's important that you learn to recognize the difference between an approach or set of techniques grounded in evidence that you can use to inform your practice and an "innovation" that is making someone a lot of money (Meichenbaum & Lilienfeld, 2018). I'm not going to name names or approaches here, mostly on the advice of my publisher's lawyers, but they're easy enough to spot; often these are based on sketchy science or are just a repackaging of some other well-established approach to treatment. Keep in mind that wherever you have a group of anxious perfectionists, there's an opportunity to exploit that anxiety for money, and there's no more obvious group of anxious perfectionists than new therapists.

In A.J. Jacobs' book *Drop Dead Healthy* (2012), he interviews Dr. Marion Nestle, a professor of nutrition, food studies, and public health and asks her about the value of superfoods like blueberries. She tells him that she doesn't believe in the concept of "superfoods"; essentially, trendy foods like quinoa, acai berries, and bone broth get all the attention but at the end of the day, the benefits are incremental beyond the basic foundations of nutrition. She explains that most of us would probably do better to get more of the boring fundamentals like apples and oranges into our diets, and then reinforces her point by ordering a plate of cream-stuffed pastries for lunch.

I think this is true for psychotherapy too. A lot of the "Great Clinical Wisdom" is already out there and most of it is free through your institution's library. Build the alliance, make therapy safe for clients, agree on goals, draw on evidence-informed practices, help clients make connections

---

1 Respectively, Acceptance & Commitment Therapy, Cognitive Behavioural Therapy, Emotion Focused Therapy, Dialectical Behavioural Therapy, and Internal Family Systems.

between their experiences, help them to find new ways of being – these have all been said in different ways by different people for over 70 years and all of these strategies work to some degree (e.g., Meier et al., 2023; Wampold, 2015). Unfortunately, there's no money to be made on this. You can't promote a new workshop or sell a book or go on talk shows touting this revolutionary new idea that clients need empathy and validation. You've got to dress it up, come up with a whole vocabulary, make up a new three-letter acronym – only then can you charge people $1,500 for the introductory workshop and launch your empire of three-letter-acronym-practicing therapists. Watch out for hype, branding, and fads; instead, try to stick with the apples and oranges of therapy. I promise you'll be just as successful, and you'll save yourself the $1,500.

Working with silence

A lot of beginner therapists talk too much, which is completely normal and probably unavoidable. I think it's a combination of two issues. (1) A lot of people tend to babble when they're nervous, and new therapists are almost always nervous, and (2) we spend an entire degree teaching you stuff that you should *do* and *say* to help heal your clients, but there's rarely a "Using silence in the clinical setting" class. We spend hardly any time talking about stuff not to do: when to leave something alone, when to back off, and how to just shut up when necessary. But silence can be extremely powerful. In a world that values talking and creating and doing (Cain, 2012), sitting back and leaving space can be enormously effective.

Years ago, I was working at a prison and my client did not want to be seeing me for therapy at all, but his treatment team was insisting that this happen. As you might guess, folks who have been mandated, pushed, or otherwise coerced into treatment tend not to be the most willing to cooperate (McGuinness et al., 2013; Snyder & Anderson, 2009) so the adoption of this attitude on his part was wholly expected and probably fair under the circumstances. This client was manifesting his unhappiness by not saying much during our meetings. My supervisor on the case challenged me to use the power of silence to my advantage.

Supervisor: How long do you think you could stay silent before getting uncomfortable?
Me: About a minute?
Supervisor: Why don't you try leaving 5 minutes of silence in your next session?

My supervisor could not have issued a more awkward or difficult challenge, but I trusted him so I decided to give it a go. In the very next session, when my client fell into his usual pattern of stonewalling me, I decided that this was a good moment to just sit in the silence he was creating. Time stretched, and neither of us said anything. The client stared at me defiantly. I stared back, hoping to visually demonstrate that therapeutically effective mixture of empathy and assertiveness. The second hand on the wall clock began to slow and go backwards as time itself began to warp. I decided to casually get my water bottle out and nonchalantly take a sip to show just how comfortable I was with the silence, that I was not the least bit disconcerted by the client's stance. I got the bottle out, twisted the cap... and nothing happened. It was stuck. I tightened my grip and tried again. No dice. Now I was truly vexed. The client was still staring at me, no one had said a word in at least two whole minutes, and my casual attempt to occupy the space wasn't working. I was not about to be defeated by a recalcitrant water bottle; I squeezed until I'm sure my eyeballs bulged like a cartoon rabbit and finally got the damn thing open. This victory gave me the lift I needed to make it through at least another minute, at which juncture I felt my point had been made and resumed the verbal portion of our session. Yes, the client won the actual stand-off, but I believe I had the moral victory.

The point of this story is twofold. (1) Therapy offers unparalleled opportunities to make an ass of yourself and (2) you never know what will move into the space you create. Clients may bring something up that you've not heard before. They may connect the dots between a couple of seemingly disparate issues. They may use the space to let themselves feel something that they've been trying to avoid, or they may just take a minute to breathe and centre themselves. If you're as uncomfortable as I was, practice silence in role plays with your colleagues or supervisors. Importantly, figure out where you're going to look during that time; you don't want to stare aggressively at your client but neither do you want to be looking out the window. Take those minutes to consider the therapy session so far and what you might want to do with the remaining time.

Give silence a whirl, I'll wait. Quietly.

Learn from everything and everyone

I was watching the show *Bluey* the other day with my toddler. For the uninitiated, *Bluey* is an animated Australian television program about a family of anthropomorphic dogs; surprisingly, it is chock-full of life lessons and therapeutic wisdom. In this episode, Bingo (the youngest child) is granted three "dance mode" cards as an apology from her father, who took her last French fry without asking. A "dance mode" card allows the bearer to insist that the target dance at any time, in any place. Unfortunately for Bingo, everyone else in the family keeps taking her dance mode cards; even though she agrees every time, it's made clear from non-verbals that she isn't really okay giving them away. At the end of the episode, Mum says to Bingo "Sometimes, does your outside voice say 'yes' when your inside voice says 'no'?" In all my time as a clinician, I have never heard boundaries explained so clearly and so succinctly, in a way that even a child could understand. Pure poetry! Note that the story ends happily: Bingo gets to make her parents dance in front of a large crowd in a public space, which seems like a harsh but fair penalty.

I used to feel guilty about borrowing lines or ideas from non-therapy sources like television shows or novels. I thought that most of what I said in therapy should come from books, lectures, or workshops; at the very least, it should be cite-able in American Psychological Association (APA) format. The turning point for me came when I described a piece of therapy wisdom that seemed appropriate to my client to my clinical supervisor that I had originally heard from a TV show. I thought the therapist had made an astute and well-worded observation but I felt uncomfortable using a line from television in therapy (it was a cheesy '90s drama). She pointed out to me that even though the line was spoken by an actress, it was created by a writer, meaning that the line ultimately came from another human based on their life experiences and those around them. I felt a lot of freedom going forward from that moment to integrate both formal and informal sources of knowledge into my work.

True clinical wisdom can come from anywhere. If a line from television or a movie or a song or a book resonates with you, use it. One of the purposes of art is to better understand the human experience, and I think psychotherapy is poorer when we don't consider the world outside of randomized control trials and textbooks. As Bluey (the heroine of *Bluey*) once said, "I don't want a valuable life lesson, I just want an ice cream." Okay, maybe that line's not relevant to this discussion but it's still true in many situations.

Opportunities to implement learning come back around

Once upon a time, I saw a young Black woman for disordered eating. I did my best to assess and treat her, but I wasn't satisfied with the outcome of that case. I had the nagging sense that I could have gone a lot further in understanding the antecedents of her symptoms and how they interacted with one another. Three weeks later, I found myself sitting across the room from another young Black woman with eerily similar patterns of disordered eating. I'm not a Jungian by any means but it certainly felt like synchronicity (Jung, 1960), and I was actually able to implement some of the lessons I had learned from the previous client. This has happened a number of times over the years where I've had two clients in relatively quick succession with strangely similar demographic characteristics and symptom profiles. Is it synchronicity? Is it just coincidence? Does Freud's ghost keep watch over our caseloads and send us the clients we need to further our development? Who knows, but it happens routinely.

The corollary to all this, of course, is that even when you do learn lessons and are able to do things differently with your second chance, a good outcome is still not guaranteed. I once saw an anxious middle-aged man with narcissistic personality features, and I'm ashamed to say that I lost my temper in session and confronted the client in a way that was not at all clinically useful. He never came back to therapy, which is totally understandable. A few weeks later, I saw another anxious middle-aged man with narcissistic personality features. This time, I vowed not to lose my temper and to maintain an empathic, non-confrontational stance no matter how much I felt provoked. I really can't say whether I was much more successful with that second client, but I can say that I felt happier with my own approach. Sometimes feeling more satisfied with your own performance can be your chief metric for conceptualizing improvement. Or, in other words, you'll sleep better at night knowing you did your best.

Real-life clients sound nothing like textbook clients

I love therapy textbooks – they're one of my favourite genres of fiction. The dialogues between therapist and client are so beautiful, so perfect, so effortless. They typically go something like this:

Client: Sometimes my coworker really gets on my nerves.
Therapist: That sounds frustrating. What would happen if you tried explaining non-judgmentally what you find irritating and asking him nicely to make some changes in his behaviour?
Client: I don't know. I suppose I could give it a try.
Therapist: Do you want to practice in session?
Client: Sure!

Here's how I see that dialogue unfolding in real therapy sessions:

Client: Sometimes my coworker really gets on my nerves.
Therapist: That sounds frustrating. What would happen if you tried explaining non-judgmentally what you find irritating and asking him nicely to make some changes in his behaviour?
Client: He'd be a total jerk about it, like he is about everything.

Therapist: Wow. It must be so tough to work with someone who has that attitude. What if we tried practicing being more assertive together in session?

Client: That would never work because he's such a complete tool.

Earlier in my career, I found the discrepancy between the dialogues presented in my textbooks and the ones I had with real-life clients very disheartening. I was concerned that my sometimes-clumsy verbiage was impeding my clients' progress; correspondingly, I believed that if I could just memorize the right set of words or the perfect phrasing, delivered with the perfect intonation, I could unlock powerful changes in my clients. I now understand that it's not all about me. There's no magic word or sentence or even group of sentences that can trigger behaviour change, primarily because behaviour is just very hard to change. It takes time and a whole lot of different words from different people to help someone see what they need to do, how to do it, and, most importantly, feel ready to do it. Textbooks are designed to represent best-case scenarios and idealized explanations; the authors are trying to neatly illustrate the concepts they're describing, and they don't have the time or space to illustrate every possible response you might get from a real client.

The real world is a lot messier but it's also a whole lot more fun. The dialogue above was inspired by a client I once saw who did have a problem with their coworker. We discussed assertive communication strategies and we talked about potential barriers to their implementation. In the following session, I checked in to see whether they had done their assigned homework.

Here's the textbook version of that conversation:

Me: Were you able to calmly and respectfully ask your colleague to respect your boundaries?

Client: It was difficult, but I communicated with her assertively and it went surprisingly well. Our interactions at work have been so much smoother as a result!

Me: How wonderful!

And here's what actually happened:

Me: Were you able to calmly and respectfully ask your colleague to respect your boundaries?

Client: No, I went all "Animal Planet" on her ass instead. There was so much screaming the manager ended up sending us both home.

To this day, I can't help but think of "going Animal Planet" on someone as the polar opposite of calm, respectful communication. Your clients won't usually sound like textbooks, but there's a lot of charm to real, authentic exchanges with a client who obviously trusts you enough to share the unvarnished truth. I don't see a lot of laughter or humour in therapy textbooks, but I have seen a lot of it in my therapy rooms. I prefer the latter.

When clients don't seem to be making progress

The course of therapy is rarely straightforward. In my entire career, I think I've had about two clients who came in, shared their clear, well-defined issues, did their homework consistently, saw linear improvement, and terminated in a neat manner. Every other therapy experience I've had has been much more convoluted: clients' symptoms get worse, their progress stalls out, they get stuck and feel frustrated with their situations. They're not bad clients and you're not a bad therapist, it's just the natural complexity of their problems. Therapy parallels life, and life is more of a "two steps forward, one step back" kind of experience, or sometimes it's "four steps backward, two steps forward, one step backward, three steps forward" with a couple of diagonal and sideways steps thrown in. You get it.

I was working with a client who had very challenging symptoms towards the end of graduate school. They were a student with perfectionistic tendencies who couldn't get anything done because every word in every sentence in every assignment for every course had to be absolutely, completely perfect before they could move on. A single paragraph could take a week, and one page of an essay could take a month; as a result, they were in their 40s and still desperately trying to complete an undergraduate degree. My first strategy was to tackle the perfectionism symptoms directly, but the client was not interested in exposure-based approaches. Okay, no problem. We switched to addressing the unhelpful thoughts and beliefs driving the behaviour. No dice. Then we refocused treatment goals on the client's procrastination. Again, very little movement. From there, we moved on to the sleep problems that were impairing their ability to concentrate on the writing. When that didn't work, we targeted the stressful marriage, that was impairing their sleep, that was fuelling the procrastination, that drove the perfectionism that caught the cat, that ate the rat, that lived in the house that Jack built! Round and round we went but in months of work, the client saw hardly any progress at all and began to express frustration with therapy. I became very disheartened and started to lose hope.

One afternoon, I poured out my concerns to my supervisor, Doug, and he offered to share with me the secret to making progress in psychotherapy when clients seem to be stuck. "My goodness," I thought. "The secret that will fix this situation! The secret that will set me and the client free from this miserable, stressful cycle! The fix that will deliver us both from multiple months of hell!" I leaned in, pen poised over notebook, breathless with anticipation. "Don't let them be the last client you see in a day," said Doug, and sat back, smiling at me genially. After that build-up, I wanted to smack him. "Don't let them be the last client?!" What kind of garbage advice was this? I wanted to make this person better, not optimize my schedule.

Some clients will not experience improvements with therapy – up to one third, depending on where you work (Howard et al., 1986; Lambert, 2013). A proverb I've heard repeated among clinicians is "Don't work harder than your clients," which is the psychotherapy spin on "You can lead a horse to water, but you can't make them drink." Fundamentally, working harder than your clients just doesn't work: you can't "fix" your clients by pouring in your own time and energy because improvement is ultimately up to them and the changes they feel able to make. More than likely, the result is likely to be nagging on your part, followed quickly by resentment on their part, and possibly some level of shutting down in both of you. And nobody wins when therapy gets to that point.

Whether or not your clients improve, it's crucial that you don't burn out from working with clients who are presently stuck or who have more challenging presenting issues. You don't want to spend your evenings and weekends re-evaluating your life choices just because three sessions went well and the last one was mediocre. To be honest, I still try too hard all too often even though life has shown me time and time again that sometimes, sitting back is what I really need to do. However, I do make it a point not to end my day with clients that are struggling to make progress.

It's okay if your work isn't a calling

There's a prevailing belief that if you've gone into a helping profession, this is your calling. You're not just a therapist by training, it's your identity: you are a Helper. I find this way of thinking concerning for a couple of different reasons.

Firstly, being in a helping profession doesn't have to be a professional calling in order for you to do good work. You can work hard in your program, care about your clients' well-being, be an ethical practitioner, and still see it as a job. Viewing this work as a satisfactory way to pay your bills does not automatically imply that you'll be phoning it in or doing a lacklustre job. For example, I'd wager that most of us don't know if our dentist sees their work as a calling, but we trust them anyway. In fact, there may be moments in your professional life where this perspective is an asset: if you experience setbacks or difficulties or even just professional doldrums, you may be upset but you won't necessarily see the situation as a threat to your whole identity.

Secondly, once a particular job is seen as a "calling," this belief can be used by unscrupulous politicians, managers, or CEOs to justify treating people in that job very poorly. Think of nursing or teaching, two jobs very commonly seen as "callings" and two jobs that pay very poorly relative to the demands of the work (Britton & Propper, 2016; Chang et al., 2019). If we believe that people will stay in a job no matter what because it's "who they are," it then becomes much easier to restrict raises, cut back on their benefits, and otherwise compromise their job security. It also means that the people in those jobs may be socialized to tolerate all kinds of abuse and poor behaviour from the populations with whom they work, which shouldn't be the case in any job.

That being said, it's also very much okay if you do see psychotherapy as a calling and can't imagine your life going in any other direction. Congratulations to you on identifying and pursuing such a meaningful goal! Hold on to that perspective because it will probably help get you through tough times. But don't stop advocating for your profession – just because you've landed your dream job and will spend the rest of your life working in it doesn't mean you shouldn't get a great pension when you're ready to retire and sick leave when you need it.

Conclusion

Whether your journey through graduate school is short or long, there's going to be lots of ups and downs. One minute, you'll feel like you're finally getting the hand of things and might even be helping your clients, the next it'll seem like you're back at the beginning, completely unsure and unprepared as you start work at a new setting or with a new client. This is uncomfortable but it's definitely normal. Just like your clients, your journey to improvement probably won't be linear but that's okay – if this was easy, everybody would be doing it. Just remind yourself that you did eventually get the hang of driving (even on highways!) and you'll figure this one out too.

Chapter 3

Supervisee

Most training programs in psychotherapy require students to participate in a mysterious activity called "clinical supervision." My program prepared us well for this by giving us a comprehensive and detailed manual explaining the function and purpose of supervision, as well as the role of the supervisor and the supervisee, typical content of supervision, common pitfalls, professional behaviour in supervision, and clear directives about who to approach with problems. Oh no, wait...that was just a beautiful dream I had. Instead, they sent me an email saying, "Report to Dr. Smith for supervision on Thursday at 5pm." At the appointed hour, I dutifully joined a group of students of varying degree of seniority and sat quietly in a conference room while trying to get the lay of the land, completely unsure whether I would be required to speak and what I would say should that happen. It was nerve-wracking to say the least.

For those of you whose training programs took a similar approach to mine, let's review the basics of clinical supervision. When you start to see your own clients independently, a "grown-up" therapist (i.e., someone with a license) will keep a close eye on what you're doing and how; this is to provide guidance, direction, and overall oversight as they assume the ultimate legal and ethical responsibility for the case. Supervision comes in a variety of formats including one-on-one and in a group with other students; common activities include discussing the case, watching videos/audio of sessions, problem-solving, resolving ethical issues and learning about different presenting issues and client groups. You are likely to address overall goals with the client, content to explore in session, assessments to do and interventions to deliver, and management of the therapeutic alliance. In an ideal world, this person will support both your clinical and professional development.

But all of that is just the official story. Let's dive into how things really get done.

DOI: 10.4324/9781003355366-5

Preparing for supervision

Supervision is intended to offer you the chance to learn, to practice new skills, and to make mistakes in a safe context (Bailin et al., 2018; Borders et al., 2023); to maximize your learning opportunities and get the most out of this, you need to be open, honest, and receptive to feedback (Falender & Shafranske, 2017; Parker et al., 2017). This is much easier said than done, but you can stack the deck by preparing. Before you arrive to your first supervision session, think about what you need at this point in your training to facilitate your own learning and development, and what you require from your supervisor to successfully implement their recommendations and make changes. If you're new to supervision, think back to other situations in your life where you regularly received constructive criticism, like school or work. Who gave you useful feedback and what worked about how they delivered it? Think back also to your less-good experiences receiving feedback (apologies, I know no one likes this type of reminiscing) to figure out what *didn't* work and why? Think about issues like the timing of feedback delivery, the balance between positive and negative comments, and the impact of doing all this within a group context, if this is the case in your training site. For example, I generally need time to digest and reflect on someone's comments and manage my emotional reaction to the news before I respond to them; therefore, a major pet peeve of mine in graduate school was when supervisors expected me to respond to their feedback immediately and on the spot.

If you can, try to have a chat with your supervisor about their philosophy and approach to supervision before you start working together. What's their style, what's your style, and how can you mesh those effectively? Before you start, ask other students who have worked with that person how it went and what they most liked and disliked. Hopefully what you hear makes you feel confident and eager to start ("Dr. Ménard is fantastic!"). However, if it doesn't ("Dr. Ménard is a major hard-ass and she's obsessed with paperwork!"), start thinking about how you could adjust to manage the situation. Keep in mind also that fit is important, and you may have a different experience with this person than other students (see below). No matter how supervision goes, the experience will be useful. With fantastic supervisors, you can try to emulate their best qualities in your own practice, and with less-than-ideal supervisors, you'll know what not to do yourself down the road.

Supervision can be hard

Clinical supervision can be a very challenging part of your training. You're learning a brand-new set of skills, and part of that learning involves meeting with an expert in that area, sharing everything you did, and then receiving feedback about what to do differently. Learning *any* new set of skills can be nerve-wracking, and this is a particularly difficult set of skills: the learning curve is very intense, particularly at the beginning, and you will likely be sharing a lot of mistakes and missteps. Every supervisor also has their own sometimes weird, sometimes persnickety way of doing things (isn't persnickety a fun word?). One supervisor's perfect note may be another's rough draft. One supervisor may want to review your therapy tapes at every meeting and another may never do it ever. Getting the hang of what someone is looking for can take a while, and as soon as you figure that out, you'll be on to a new supervisor.

Add to this already-challenging scenario is the fact that most supervisors don't receive formal training in clinical supervision (Watkins Jr., 2012). This is something of a personal peeve for me as most psychologists do end up providing supervision at some point in their careers (Barnett, 2017), yet few of us are taught to do it; I worry the same is true in the other helping professions. Imagine learning to cook by trying to identify what went wrong with the worst meals you've ever had and comparing that with what went right in the best ones! Anyway, until the world of clinical training comes to its senses and starts doing things my way, you can guess that the person overseeing your case may have cobbled together their approach over time and experience, which may produce inconsistent results.

Always keep in mind that providing clinical supervision is like watching a tennis game and coaching the player. You're the one who's actually on the court, running round, trying to return shots, making sure you don't commit fouls, and whatever else tennis involves (note to my editor: should I just stay away from sports metaphors altogether?). I've been both the player and the coach a lot over the years and at least for me, supervising a case is much easier than being the clinician in the room. You've got the harder job – feel free to remind yourself of this whenever you feel your supervisor is being annoying.

Be yourself but also push yourself

> Between the ages of twenty and forty we are engaged in the process of discovering who we are, which involves learning the differences between accidental limitations which it is our duty to outgrow and the necessary limitations of our nature beyond which we cannot trespass with impunity
>
> (W.H. Auden, *The Dyer's Hand*, 1962)

To me, this quotation embodies the ethos of good supervision, which should be a marvelous opportunity to discover who you are as a clinician.

What aspects of your clinical self are fundamental parts of who you are and what parts should you grow and change? Where do you need to stretch, explore, expand, or get out of your comfort zone?

Hopefully you will have the opportunity to be supervised by lots of different types of therapists: people of different theoretical orientations, people with different approaches to assessment or intervention, people with markedly different clinical styles. Try on facets of their approach while they supervise you to see what fits and what doesn't. If you're someone who naturally gravitates to CBT, hone your EFT skills with a supervisor who has trained in this approach. If you like very structured sessions, let your supervisor guide you through a more unstructured approach. If you don't like using exercises or worksheets in session, take the chance to learn how to do this, then decide later if you ever want to do this again. Similarly, your supervisor may sometimes make a recommendation with which you disagree: an area to assess further, a type of intervention to implement or a clinical skill to deploy. Attending clinical supervision is, in many ways, an act of faith; try to set aside your doubt and give it a shot. You might think that neither you nor the client will get anything out of it, but you might be surprised. The worst that can happen is that it's not a good fit and you don't incorporate a strategy into your practice permanently, and the best that can happen is that you learn something about yourself as a practitioner that you didn't know before. I've often used a version of this with clients: "Try this homework and if it doesn't work, come back and tell me that I was totally wrong and this was a bad suggestion." I can't tell you how many clients perk up at the chance to tell their therapist they're wrong. The same is true for the students I supervise – I request that they try something new, but if it fails, they are free to editorialize when they give me their feedback. But I do ask them to give it a try first.

Recently, a grad student in my supervision group was struggling with "resting sarcastic voice," a rare condition conceptually related to "resting bitch face" but centred on her default tone of voice: she frequently sounded sarcastic even when she had no intention to be. As a result, her attempts to congratulate the client on progress and accomplishments sounded flat and muted at best. We identified this as an area for growth and I encouraged her to find her inner cheerleader and muster as much enthusiasm as she could in session. She embraced the challenge with vigour, ultimately using our class time to practice on her fellow students: "Way to go, Matt!! You did an excellent job sharing your case conceptualization!!" By the end of the semester, she had found more energy for her clinical praise, but in a way that was still authentic to her personality. By contrast, I might be a little *too* enthusiastic in my delivery of praise: most recently, my toddler successfully stacked three blocks one on top of the other and I cheered so hard that I startled her. I probably need to practice toning it down – maybe in group supervision with the other moms.

To each their own supervisor

In my first external placement at a hospital, my principal supervisor was very terse; in retrospect, I'm guessing that she was over-worked and under-paid relative to her responsibilities. Most of that placement involved me observing while she conducted structured diagnostic interviews and then we'd spend a short time afterwards identifying the Diagnostic and Statistical Manual (DSM-IV-TR) diagnoses for which that person qualified. I will say that she helped me to understand the diagnostic criteria for severe mental illness better than anyone I have worked with, but I thought she fell short in providing guidance on the process or content of assessment and intervention more broadly. I also did not in any way associate this person with any degree of warmth or fuzziness. One fine day, a few months after I'd started, a client I had seen for a few sessions of therapy on the inpatient unit took an overdose of medication and was taken to the emergency room. As I had seen them for an appointment just that morning, I was terrified and felt that I must have dramatically screwed up in some way. How could I have failed to notice their state of mind and intervene? Was I the worst student to ever set foot in that hospital? My supervisor and I went to the file room to carefully double-check the paperwork in this client's file and update it. A psychiatrist who was in the room working on his own charts decided this was the perfect moment to make a deeply unfunny "joke" about how my session must have driven the client to their overdose. My not-warm, not-fuzzy supervisor snapped back at him with the ferocity of a bulldog and he meekly clammed up and went back to charting with his head down. I don't think he spoke to me directly for the rest of my placement. Many years later, this is my chief memory of her: protective of her student when it counted. This moment may also represent the start of my life-long grudge towards the entire subspecialty of psychiatry.

Within supervisory relationships, one person's hard-ass is another person's ferocious defender and conversely, one student's non-directive jellyfish might be the gentle corrective experience another student desperately needs. It may take you a few different supervisors to figure out what works best for you, what you like and don't like, where you need the most help and what you need that help to look like, but it's worth taking the time to think it through as this can help you ask for what you need in future supervisory relationships. Similar to the client–therapist relationship, the fit in supervisory relationships may vary significantly (Barnett & Molzon, 2014; Falender & Shafranske, 2014; Watkins Jr., 2017); this is just the nature of human personalities, and not a reflection on the skills or qualities of either person. Some pairings will be amazing, life-enhancing opportunities for both supervisor and supervisee, some will be absolutely awful, and most will be somewhere in the middle. Not every supervisor–student match is going to produce the magic of Mr. Miyagi and the karate kid (yes, this is from the 1984 movie, *The Karate Kid*, and yes, I'm dating myself). Do feel free to question the supervisory skill of anyone who expects you to wax their car during a training experience, though, as that definitely shouldn't be happening.

Reach out to senior students

I'm not saying that all your professors are out-of-touch relics who probably got their clinical training when dinosaurs roamed the earth, but I also don't know how to finish this sentence truthfully. Let's start over. In a lot of cases, supervisors have been in the field for so long that they've forgotten what it was like to not have their clinical knowledge and skills. They don't remember a time when they didn't speak the language of therapy, or when their heads weren't filled with all the information that you're now desperately trying to cram into yours. You know who remembers well your current state of mixed anxiety-excitement-eagerness? The students in the years directly above you, and they'll be able to speak to you at your level. They are a valuable resource so use them! If you want to get fancy, we could call this peer supervision and there's a lot of research showing the benefits of this approach (Basa, 2019; Golia & McGovern, 2015; Nelson, 2014). Reach out, make a coffee date, and bring your list of questions. "What's the best way to introduce this intervention?" or "I forgot what this part of the thought record is meant to capture!" or "How do you stay on top of your paperwork?" And maybe buy their coffee for them as a thank you.

You know your client, your supervisor knows that type of problem

As a graduate student, I often felt frustrated at my supervisors when I thought their recommendations were misplaced. Assess this issue further? I already know what's going on in that area of the client's life. Focus more on emotions than cognitions in session? I don't think that'll work with this fellow. Speak slower in therapy? Um, that suggestion was pretty on the nose, but I've really only got the one talking speed (a squirrel on cocaine). I would sit in supervision and fret that the supervisor had only heard my descriptions of the case – how could they understand the nuances of the situation when they'd not been in the room with the client themselves? If they had, they would surely see it my way.

With the wisdom of hindsight and many years of experience as a supervisor myself, I can now confidently say that I was right, but so were all of my supervisors. This particular lesson came home to me sharply after I had become a supervisor myself at a hospital. It was our regular practice to provide clients who were seen on the inpatient unit details about our clinic's outpatient services and encourage them to follow up with us for psychotherapy after they were discharged; however, it was a very, very rare occurrence that any client did and I learned quickly not to expect them back no matter what polite assurances they made before they left. But every year, the new incoming students would push back, swearing to me, "I shared the information and the client promised he'd call after he's discharged." And then I'd give them the kind of knowing smile that supervisors spend hours perfecting alone in the bathroom and say not-at-all condescendingly, "I'm sure he will."

You, the clinician, are definitely the expert on your particular client because of the hours you've spent together, but your supervisor is the expert on patterns of behaviour across many clients and they may be less likely to get distracted by the details. Both forms of knowing are valuable but when in doubt, consider your supervisor's perspective. Trust that they've made most if not all the mistakes and missteps that can be made in therapy and that their sage guidance is designed to prevent you from doing the same.

My classmates are all doing better than me (and other cognitive distortions)

My earliest clinical supervision experiences were almost entirely in group format; theoretically, we were all new to the process of assessing and intervening with clients but practically, some of my classmates seemed to be leaps and bounds ahead of me. Sarah effortlessly led her client through empty-chair exercises, Rebecca deftly navigated ethical dilemmas with a complex case, Emma knew exactly what interventions to implement and when…I felt like the only one in the room struggling with all those things. Predictably, this made attending group supervision rather unpleasant – I don't know about you, but I don't do my best learning when I'm wrapped in a thick layer comprised of equal parts self-doubt and envy.

In hindsight, I suspect that we were all struggling in different areas, but I just couldn't see it at the time. As a clinical supervisor, I have the benefit of (1) experience with a lot of different students and (2) a higher-level view. In a group setting, I can look out over the room of students and see everyone's strengths and areas for improvement. Some students do well forming therapeutic alliances but have difficulty explaining interventions to clients, others excel at writing therapy notes but need help making the connections required for a thorough case conceptualization, and some students readily grasp and implement supervisory feedback while others may need several meetings to understand the nuances of the recommendation. I have yet to meet a student who is naturally good at every single piece of the rich tapestry that makes up clinical work.

Even if you can't see where others are struggling, know that they are because therapy is a tough skill to master. You have areas for further growth and development and so do they, I promise. Likewise, if you become totally fixated on everyone else's strengths but can't see your own, know that you have them. Ask your supervisor what you're doing well and practice looking for the evidence yourself. To summarize: if you believe your classmates are all doing better than you, no they aren't.

Speak up, part 1

Late in my own graduate training, I was providing peer supervision to a more junior student who was working with a client who had symptoms of social anxiety. "So you'll want to create a fear hierarchy with them in the next session and then explain about avoidance and safety behaviours because you want to make sure they don't interfere with the exposure exercises…" I was sailing along in my little speech when the student interrupted: "I know what a fear hierarchy is but how exactly do I go about creating one with the client? What do I actually say in session?" My rant screeched to a halt abruptly. "Good point!" I said, "Let's do a little role play and then you can use the same strategy with your client to generate examples that are meaningful to them."

Therapy is a language onto itself. Think "Fear hierarchy", "activity scheduling", "contingency management", or "grounding exercises"; I still giggle when I get to say "exposure." When you first start learning therapy, there's a whole wide world of terminology that is likely brand-new to you. Sure, you've read these terms in books but there's a difference between seeing something on the page and actually doing the activity yourself.

If you forget something, if you don't know what a word means, if you don't know how to introduce or facilitate a specific exercise in therapy, speak up! Ask your supervisor to spell out the nitty-gritty of how to do something. If you're anxious or embarrassed, here's a good linguistic cheat: "Remind me, what does [X] mean?" The "remind me" implies that of course you know, you just need a brief refresher. Similarly, you can ask for a supervisor's personal recommendation on how to implement a specific exercise. "How do *you* like to introduce a thought record?" Again, this implies that you know perfectly well how to do the task, but you're interested in their specific perspective. Keep in mind that in a group supervision setting, you are undoubtedly not the only person with that question and other students might benefit from the review themselves. It doesn't matter how many times you've read about a term or had it explained to you – you're trying to master an enormous amount of information all at once and it's natural that some things are going to slip through the cracks. You just need a little reminder.

Speak up, part 2

Life is what happens while you're busy doing graduate school. It seems unjust that you don't get a break while you're doing all this extra training to be a certified Good Person who helps other people with their troubles but difficult circumstances may arise in your life during this time. You may find yourself confronting sudden and unexpected issues during your clinical training like car accidents, financial catastrophes, relationship breakdowns, illness (pet or human), or the loss of loved ones. If you think it's likely to affect some aspect of your clinical functioning, whether that's scheduling and attending sessions, completing paperwork, handling administrative issues, responding to communications in a timely manner, attending supervision, or anything else, let your supervisor know as soon as possible. You don't have to be specific about the details but share the general contours of the issue: how long it's likely to persist, which areas of your work are likely to be affected, and how they can help. Even if the explanation is "An awful thing is happening, I don't know how long it's going to last or what I'm going to do!", that's better than nothing. At this point, you and your supervisor will want to try to identify and differentiate the absolute essential elements of the work versus those that can be put on the back-burner until life calms down just a smidge. At one site, I had a supervisee share that their partner had been involuntarily hospitalized for psychiatric issues and there was no knowing whether their stay was likely to be a few days or a few months. This was definitely a new challenge for both of us and hard to plan around, but at least we were on the same page. I wasn't surprised or upset when the student was late to work several times over the following weeks and needed a little more support in supervision meetings.

Part of professional development is figuring out how to manage the job during times of stress (see also Chapter 5); if you have a chance to get some guidance while you're still under supervision, that can be the silver lining to your otherwise terrible situation. Most people are better prepared to respond to potential problems and emergencies with a little bit of forewarning and supervisors are no exception.

Your supervisors are human

I'm breaking the supervisor code to admit this, but we're all flawed. We've all made clinical mistakes, even if we don't openly share them. We weren't born knowing how to administer an intelligence test or explain a thought record or create the perfect case conceptualization. Hopefully, you'll have supervisors who share some of their goofs with you because, at the end of the day, supervisors are really just slightly older grad students with a few more layers of experience (and the white hairs that come with them). I try to walk that fine line between sharing enough of my mistakes with students for them to know I'm human, but not so many that they think I'm just plain incompetent at my job.

As humans, your supervisors may let you down. Occasionally, this might mean they forget something, like a meeting or paperwork to review. Sometimes they might try to rush you through a discussion when you'd like a little more time to process or give you feedback that's too vague to be useful. They might tell you to add a sentence in a report and then tell you in the next set of revisions to take it out (I call this report-writing hokey-pokey – you put the sentence in, you take the sentence out, you put the sentence back in, and you shake it all about). All of these issues are fixable: send reminders to absent-minded supervisors and be as assertive and proactive as you can about your needs.

Sometimes the rupture might be more serious. One of my favourite supervisors in graduate school was Doug – you may recall that he helped me manage a case that was causing me a lot of stress (see Chapter 2, p. 32). He taught me so much about diagnosis, treatment, and foundational clinical skills. He was supportive of my professional development and a gifted clinician; I still use many of his lessons in training students myself. A decade after our work together ended, I found out that he lost his license after getting into a sexual relationship with someone he was seeing for psychotherapy. Even though I hadn't worked with him for quite some time, I still felt confused and hurt – it was so hard to reconcile this flagrantly unethical behaviour with the person I had known. How could he display such poor judgement? Were all his lessons and advice on other subjects completely worthless? How could I reconcile this shocking behaviour with the warm feelings I still held towards him? The answers to these questions were, respectively, "it's a shockingly common behaviour" (Lamb et al., 2003; Pope et al., 1986; Vesentini et al., 2022), "no", and "seek supervision."

At some point in the supervisee phase of your training, your supervisor will probably disappoint you in some big or small way. Try to embody that golden rule principle and extend the same grace to them as you would have them extend to you for your mistakes because even good, well-meaning supervisors make mistakes. But, just to reiterate, don't have sex with your clients. Ever. Under any circumstances. Just…no.

Addressing and managing disconnects in supervision

Over your training and career, you are likely to have multiple clinical supervisors. Some may be an amazing fit, the exact right person you need at the exact right time; others may not be such a great fit, or possibly the right person but at the wrong time. When you realize that there's a disconnect in supervision or some friction happening, try to keep perspective: it is much more likely that both you and your supervisor are good people who are confused and unsure of how to meet one another's needs rather than the world's worst student and/or the world's worst supervisor. If you can, figure out what you need to be different; you may find that talking it out with other students helps. The next step is to ask for those changes assertively, politely, and respectfully: "I've noticed that in 'X' situation, we tend to 'Y' but I'm wondering if we could give 'Z' a try instead. I've found that approach very helpful to me in other supervision settings." Make sure that what you are requesting falls within the realm of ethical and professional clinical behaviour rather than "I've noticed that when I don't get my notes done, you get irritated at me and I'm wondering if you could give me a month or two for each of them." That's just not going to happen. Try also to be specific in your requests: "Could you be less of a jerk?" is too vague to be actionable, especially if your supervisor really is a jerk.

Sometimes the issues will be a lack of fit, either in clinical approach or just in personality. It might also be the case that your needs as a supervisee have changed over time since you started your training (Barnett & Molzon, 2014; Falender & Shafranske, 2012). When you first start out, you may need a lot of guidance on what to do, and how to do it. Over time, your clinical spidey-sense will start to kick in and you'll need less concrete direction; you'll be able to spend supervision addressing subtleties in clients' presentations, challenging cases, and professional development. Some supervisors do better with different stages of clinical training than others, and that could be where you run into problems. If you're a real beginner and you've got a supervisor more used to dealing with clinicians at the end of their training, you might feel lost, unsupported, and in need of more structure and guidance. Conversely, I once had a supervisor towards the end of my Ph.D. who insisted on treating me as though I was a complete beginner and it eventually hurt our supervisor/supervisee relationship. I understand now that she was just being cautious but at the time, it felt as though she doubted my abilities, which didn't feel good, especially when I was struggling so much already with self-doubt.

Hopefully, you and your supervisor will be able to find a solution, but if those don't work, you may find yourself stuck, at least temporarily, in an uncomfortable situation. In that case, there's a few options to make the best of a bad situation. Try to identify something (anything!) that you're getting out of the relationship – some skill, some strategy, some chunk of clinical knowledge – and focus on how to internalize that one good thing. Check in with peers regularly to debrief. Do your self-care, whatever that looks like for you (see Chapter 5). Talk to other supervisors in your program – not about the specific details of the case as that remains your supervisor's responsibility but about general clinical issues relevant to your work with that client. For example: "Dr. Ménard, can you help me get the hang of explaining cognitive defusion to clients?" Give yourself preparation time and decompression time before and after supervision meetings and find ways to reaffirm your value as a clinician, if you're not getting that feedback from your supervisor. And know that if nothing else, you're getting valuable experience about what you'll try to avoid doing as a supervisor yourself down the line.

Session recording

Depending on your setting, supervision may be primarily verbal: you tell the story of the session and ask questions, your supervisor gives you guidance and suggestions for how to direct therapy or refine certain approaches. Most studies have shown that the "story-telling" method is the most common approach to clinical supervision (Nelson, 2014; O'Donovan et al., 2011), but it may not be optimal for your learning and development. As humans, we all tend to portray ourselves in the best possible light and some of us may gloss over our bumps in the attempt (obviously, I would *never* do such a thing...).

However, in some settings, you will be able to do audio or video recording of sessions. My two recommendations if you are able: (1) rewatch all your sessions yourself before supervision and (2) show random moments from the session to your supervisor. For the first few years of my training, I rewatched all of my sessions before supervision. Yes, the sound of your own voice is aggravating; I promise, over time, you will sort of (though not quite!) get used to it. Tough it out because rewatching is a chance for you to see your whole session from a different perspective. You might catch your own little tics or identify a moment where you could have slowed down or probed further; if therapy has stalled, you may identify some cycle in which you and the client are stuck that is impeding progress. Catching your own missteps or areas for further learning leads to a much more effective use of supervision because now you can use that time to check in on areas of greater confusion or where you are genuinely lost or uncertain of what to do.

In sharing video or audio, I've found that students often want to focus on moments in the session that went really well, because they like looking good in front of me and their peers (fair). Conversely, they might choose to show rockier moments in the session because they already *know* it went badly and they know what they'd like to do differently next time – they still come out looking smart because they caught the misstep. I recommend starting at a random spot where nothing special was happening. This is the best chance to pick up on the "unknown unknowns" for your supervisor: an unnoticed verbal or physical tic, a flawed explanation, a disconnect in the alliance. Or maybe everything was truly neutral and unremarkable in that moment in the session and that's good to know as well.

In summary: watch tape as often as you can and show your supervisor the random bits as often as you can, no matter how irritating you find your own voice. Trust me, we all feel that way about recordings of our own voices.

Don't be afraid to share your knowledge

The knowledge that we fight to gain during our graduate school training is often internalized through blood, sweat, and tears (so many tears); however, by the time we become "grown-up" clinicians and supervisors, much of it may already be out of date. Sometimes this is a relatively unimportant issue like how best to do a type of statistical analysis (or at least, unimportant to me) and sometimes it is something of greater consequence, like what are the most appropriate values to guide your clinical work with diverse clients (see Chapter 10).

However, you – brand-new trainee that you are – may know lots of things your supervisors don't know. You have the latest textbooks, and maybe you've even read them. You may have attended a workshop or taken a class on the very issue most relevant to your client. You might even be doing research on that topic! Share this wisdom with your supervisor. We all need to have our knowledge updated occasionally and you might be in the perfect position to do just that. This is one of the main reasons I like teaching, because of the fresh perspectives that students bring to old, familiar topics. For example, just last week, I was explaining the limits of confidentiality for psychologists in Ontario, a list I've delivered to clients literally hundreds of times, when a student asked me a question I couldn't answer. As a result, I contacted my regulatory board and we were all enlightened by the reply.

If the opportunity comes along for you to turn the tables on your supervisor and be the smartypants in the room, take it. Everyone will come away from that a little more knowledgeable and better prepared for the work.

Supervision can be life-changing

One of my early clinical supervisors was very well-meaning in her intentions but also very hard on herself. She was quite a perfectionist and looking back, I suspect she was dealing with an inferiority complex as she was still early in her professional career. I regularly felt pretty beaten-up by her supervision and all of the students her group found ourselves in tears at one point or another. It was hard to share as openly as I should have because I didn't feel comfortable being vulnerable in that situation. To be perfectly honest, this was a low stage in my graduate training, as it took place alongside other major challenges, and I gave serious thought to leaving the program altogether.

With my very next case, my supervisor started our work together by saying: "Don't yell at your clients and don't sleep with them. You can fix pretty much everything else." To this day, it is one of the single most liberating and accurate statements I have ever heard from another clinician. Although we don't seek them out, there's actually a lot of value to directly addressing mistakes we make with clients and demonstrating how to take responsibility and make repairs without overwhelming self-judgement and criticism (Eubanks et al., 2021; Friedlander et al., 2018). More importantly, I felt safe and free in this supervision group to try different strategies and share my doubts and uncertainties without the need to self-censor because I felt everything was fixable. And it was.

It's possible that you'll meet a supervisor who will radically change your approach, or you may just retain bits and pieces. Either way, you'll be on your way to becoming a better, more complex, more interesting therapist. My clinical identity is made up of little pieces of everyone who has ever supervised me, and it gives me great pleasure to pull out little nuggets of wisdom I learned from others to share with my own clients.

Conclusion

Supervision can be one of the most difficult and challenging aspects of clinical training, but it's also the part that will make the greatest contribution to your growth as a clinician. I strongly believe that the real learning of clinical work takes place in supervision – textbooks and role plays are just no substitute for direct feedback on your actual practice with real live clients. It might seem like a cliché but you'll get out of supervision what you put in so do your best to make the effort.

Chapter 4

Internship and licensure

Many mental health training programs conclude with some kind of internship: a capstone training experience ranging from several months to a full year where you work full-time as a clinician in one or more settings, albeit still under supervision. Like most transitions, this is an exciting and overwhelming time – it's ex-whelming, if you will. After so many years of training, you are so close to being done that you can almost taste it. There will be a lot of changes to negotiate as you move into being a full-time, adequately paid, "grown-up" clinician; for starters, you're definitely going to need a lot more cardigans. On the other hand, you still have quite a few big hurdles to get through before you triumphantly traverse that finish line or drag yourself across. For many, this will also include state or province-specific licensing exams; for an unlucky few, you may still need to defend a dissertation or thesis. Hang on because you're nearly there!

Track early, track often

At some point in your professional life, you are going to need to show your work. It might be for internship applications, it might be for licensing purposes but some regulatory body or official gatekeeper is going to want to know how you've been spending your time as a trainee clinician. They'll need to know how many hours you spent providing services to clients, whether you were doing assessment or treatment, how many hours of supervision you received and in what formats, your preferred font for session notes, your shoe size, the location of the Holy Grail…You know, basic clinical accounting.

Track your hours early and track them often. I *strongly* advise you to pay for tracking software and to use it weekly, if not daily. I know that you don't have much spare change when you're in school, and I know that it seems like Excel spreadsheets will get the job done. They might, but please take it from me, as someone who spent the better part of a week trying to piece together hundreds of training hours from lists in the back

DOI: 10.4324/9781003355366-6

of notebooks, poorly constructed spreadsheets, and educated guesses, do not take this route! Think of it like the difference between triple-ply toilet paper and the see-through stuff you'll find at every gas station bathroom. Yes, it might get the job done but it won't be very pleasant and if it fails, you'll have a real mess on your hands. See if your department can cover the cost of licensing the tracking software for students, and if they don't, advocate for this through your student representatives.

Here's the really crucial part of tracking: use the software regularly. Get into the habit of logging your hours as a matter of routine. Do it before you head home, between finishing your session notes and rinsing out your hot-beverage-of-choice mug. Try not to frame tracking as an irritant because that will only increase your sense of resentment that this is just one more thing you have to do before you can go home. We don't get mad about brushing our teeth every day, we just do it (although now that I think of it, I would prefer self-cleaning teeth).

The benefits of starting your tracking early are numerous. Your count will be much more accurate, for a start, though if anyone from the Association of Psychology Postdoctoral and Internship Centers asks, my count was flawless. You'll also have a chance to troubleshoot if you don't understand how certain training experiences are captured and you won't then find yourself trying to reclassify a bunch of hours down the line because of an initial mistake in categorization. You may even start to notice trends that could help you make more informed choices about where to go next with your clinical training. You'll also have the chance to see the hours start to add up over time, which will hopefully give you a warm glow, assuming there's a part of your heart that responds to number tallies. Think of it like putting your spare change in a container; there won't be many hours to log on a day-to-day basis but over time, the hours will add up. And instead of saving up for a vacation or a puppy, you're becoming a better, more experienced therapist! And you can always buy yourself a puppy as a graduation present down the road.

Again, for those in the cheap seats at the back: track early, track often. Future you will thank past you.

Take a minute to reflect on your progress

In the summer of 2011, I was preparing to apply for my pre-doctoral internship; despite having many important tasks to accomplish in a short span of time, I still made time to whine to a friend about the nightmare that was trying to collate my clinical hours. It was taking forever, I didn't understand what I was doing, and I couldn't understand my logging "system." Did I really see five clients with the same initials at just one setting? (Answer: yes). My eyes were crossing from staring at the computer screen all day, every day for a week straight. However, my friend, also a mental health professional, absolutely ruined my pity-party by saying, "I know this is frustrating but think of how far you've come. Four years ago, you had never seen a client and now you have all this knowledge and all these skills. You're going to be an independent professional soon and that's amazing! It's so cool that you're being given the chance to review everything you've accomplished before you take the next steps." Unfortunately, after she said that, I couldn't see the task any other way – it was still a difficult job, but the accounting process took on an entirely different aura from that point onward. I was forced to confront and appreciate my own learning; to this day, it was one of the most successful cognitive reframes I've ever seen. Note: this is also a lesson in the truth that your clients may not appreciate your beautiful reframes when they're emotionally invested in self-pity, as I was.

Life doesn't often give us the chance to reflect on how much we've learned and accomplished, but applying for capstone training experiences can be one of those moments if you choose to see it in that light. Before you started the program, you didn't know anything at all about how to assess or intervene with clients and now you do. Think about all the different people you've worked with, all the groups they represent, all the problems you've tackled, all the different therapeutic approaches you've learned, and all the skills you've picked up. It's a lot to learn in such a short space of time and you did it. Kudos to you!

Also, Meghan, if you're reading this, I'm still mad that you made me a better person against my will.

Managing application stress

Completing your internship and getting licensed for independent practice are processes likely to involve long, time-consuming, highly detailed applications. These applications may require you to submit graduate and undergraduate transcripts, tabulations of all your clinical training hours, descriptions for every course and every placement you've ever completed, autobiographical statements and essays, and lovingly tailored cover letters explaining why it's always been your life's ambition to learn more about clinical psychology in Edmonton[1].

There's a special kind of stress associated with completing these applications. You're so close to being done you can probably taste it. It's the

---

1 True story: when I was applying for my pre-doctoral internship, Edmonton's brochure advertising their training experience actually included a sentence saying, "It's not as cold here as everyone says it is." My take is that if you feel the need to include a clarification of this type, it might be best just to say nothing at all.

mental equivalent of children whining "Are we there yet?!" from the back-seat on a long road trip. In addition, you are likely to be juggling these applications at the same time as you are still completing your clinical training or other major milestone projects required for your degree. After all your years of training, these applications may have a lot riding on them. I completed mine with the creeping dread lurking in the back of my mind that any mistakes I made might result in me getting tossed directly out of my internship, like Moe throwing Barney out of the bar on *The Simpsons*.

My main suggestion for stress management during the application process is to treat it as a part-time job, which is to say a third or even fourth part-time job on top of your clinical training, your research, and the rest of your academic and non-academic obligations. But to the extent that you can, set aside lots and lots of time; on the advice of a colleague, I worked only four days a week as I prepared for my licensure exams and set aside my Fridays for fun activities like completing licensure paperwork and studying for exams – I threw in the occasional dentist visit to lighten things up. I know this was an enormous privilege and I was lucky to have flexible employers but see what might be possible for you in your jobs or training settings. Even one afternoon here and there is better than giving over all of your hard-earned evenings and weekends.

Similarly, if you are thinking about planning a wedding, buying a house, having a baby, getting a puppy, or any other time-consuming-but-valuable life experience, try to ensure that this life choice doesn't overlap too much with your application, internship, and licensure process. If you feel you absolutely must go ahead with your wedding/house-buying/baby-having/ puppy acquisition, get some help. Rope in family and friends, hire professionals if you can afford them – anyone who can help take the load off. Consider also giving yourself a longer timeline so that you can complete some of these activities at your leisure – this applies mainly to wedding-planning and home-buying and less so to caring for babies and puppies, who come with their own built-in timelines.

Reach out also to your colleagues who are going through the process alongside you. Consider setting aside time to work on applications together, for the purposes of accountability, moral support, sharing information, or – break glass in case of emergency – a shoulder to cry on. Pooling information can save everyone a lot of time and headaches, and senior colleagues may be able to share their experiences, application forms, and/or study materials.

Keep in mind throughout these applications or licensing exams that the results, whether bad or good, are not a reflection on your worth as a clinician. When I was going through the match process for my pre-doctoral internship, I only got three interviews out of the 12 applications I submitted, including one application submitted to the site where I was currently doing a clinical placement; many of my colleagues had twice as many interviews. To say this was a blow to my self-esteem is putting it mildly. After months of nail-biting and hand-wringing, I ultimately matched with and then completed my internship training at the site that had been at the very top of my list from the start.

Try, if you can, to give yourself time and space to get through these last few steps as painlessly as possible. Remember, you have more value as a person and as a clinician than any application process could ever measure. Feel free to repeat this as needed to yourself and your friends.

The meta-skill of starting at a new place

Learning how to start work at a new clinical site is a skill in and of itself, a kind of a meta-skill, as it were. Every clinical setting will have its own way of doing things and its own set of rules governing everything from paperwork to the client referral process, intake procedures, appointment booking, and more. Sometimes these rules are clear, transparent, intelligible, and well-documented. Sometimes it seems more likely that the rules were chiseled onto stone tablets in the mists of time by unusually bureaucratic cavepeople and have not been revisited in the millennia since. Regardless, they are now your rules and you're going to have to figure them out.

This process of getting up to speed is likely to take a few weeks or sometimes longer as you try to absorb dozens of pieces of information in a short space of time while simultaneously carrying out your new, normal working activities. You'll need to learn new systems for paperwork, logging client information, client scheduling, payment processes, and, depending on the setting, floor plans. At one hospital job, I spent an entire lunch break doing laps around the corridors until I was confident that I knew where to find unit "5Q" if called upon to go there; you may be less directionally challenged than I am. For your first few weeks, observe your new workspace and take notes for yourself on everything; no matter how obvious something seems in the moment, I guarantee you won't remember in a few days (much like labeling containers of leftover food for the freezer). If you can identify a friendly new colleague who will answer dozens of questions and is even willing to repeat answers they've already given you, lean on them as needed and maybe buy them lunch at some point as a thank you. Administrative assistants are often a rich source of knowledge about finicky details so make friends with them early (and maintain them!).

Keep in mind that some work settings are also better and more accustomed to onboarding new clinicians than others so if you find yourself struggling, you may not be the weakest link. I've worked at some settings that had mandatory, multi-day orientation sessions with detailed information binders and name tags. Unfortunately, these are often also the same settings that onboard everyone from the psychologists to the nurses to the janitors in the same group and require all new employees to take the exact same safety quizzes during the startup process. This will probably be unhelpful as you are far more likely to get a call to help manage a client in crisis and far less likely to get a call to come clean up an unidentifiable spill. Other worksites are less accustomed to bringing on new people. I worked at one place where my boss showed me to my office and then left before identifying the location of the client files, the registration desk or the bathroom.

Most importantly: be patient with yourself. Becoming familiar with a new set of systems can be complicated and there's nothing you can do to rush it. Your colleagues won't expect you to know everything right away as long as you're making a good-faith effort to figure out the system. You will make mistakes initially that will seem positively ridiculous down the line. Checking back on my notes, I once spent the first two weeks referring to a colleague on paper as "Dr. S." when her last name actually started with an "F." Accept also that you may not be doing your absolute best work as you get adjusted not only to the new setting but possibly also to new presenting problems and client groups. That's okay too. Do your best and know that eventually, much like riding a bicycle, you'll find yourself pedalling with ease at your new setting.

Recognizing and managing impostor feelings

The first few months after finishing my degree, I went from receiving approximately six hours of supervision a week to about six hours a month. It was a big transition and I felt terrified: terrified that I was going to be allowed to see a full roster of clients with so little oversight, terrified that my private practice clients were going to expect to see some extraordinary therapeutic skills for the hourly rate they were paying, and terrified that I was going to make a horrible, unfixable mistake. My response to these feelings of fear was to use the techniques I had just spent six years mastering in graduate school: thought records, goal-setting, exposure, relaxation techniques, and mindfulness strategies. Oh, no wait – I did something much less constructive: I decided that the key to success was to read more books. I could read myself into being a better psychologist! So when I wasn't seeing clients or doing paperwork, I was reading; I probably finished a therapy book every week for a year. You may be surprised (or not) to discover that this activity did not turn me into a more relaxed, skilled, and confident independent practitioner.

The impostor phenomenon, i.e., thinking and feeling that you are not really intelligent and accomplished and that you will be discovered as a fraud (Clance & Imes, 1978; Clance, 1985), comes for most of us at some point in our training. If you haven't felt impostor feelings before, the transition to independent practice could be that moment for you; if they're already familiar friends, this might be a period of intensification. Or maybe you really are a born clinician who has always been completely self-assured in your work, in which case please use the material from this chapter to help your less-fortunate colleagues. Unfortunately, impostor feelings aren't just a nuisance; a lot of studies in academic settings (i.e., people like you) have shown that they are associated with symptoms of depression and anxiety, as well as decreased overall wellbeing and self-esteem (Ménard & Chittle, 2023).

A few years ago, I was involved in a study where we asked students to describe a time at university when they felt like an impostor (Ménard et al., 2023). We received over 800 answers, ranging from two-word answers to short essays. These results illustrated two very important issues: (1) impostor feelings are very, very common and (2) many of us feel completely alone with them. We asked students to talk about triggers for these feelings and also how they managed them. Novel experiences, like starting new jobs or new training programs, were identified by many people as a source of impostor feelings; for clinicians in training, this might include starting at new training sites or first jobs. Having high expectations for yourself was another popular trigger, which may not come as a surprise to many of you. In our study, participants described a few helpful approaches to managing impostor experiences. Some people preferred to target their emotions directly by reaching out and talking about it with friends, family, and other students, prayer or meditation, exercise of various types, and gratitude practices. Others concentrated on undermining their unhelpful impostor thoughts by focusing on self-growth, correcting irrational thoughts, building self-confidence and self-awareness, and reducing comparisons to others. Still others preferred to problem-solve their situations by setting goals, practicing, and preparing appropriately for academic challenges. All of these are constructive approaches that I would recommend. Look out for less-than-helpful approaches in yourself that might worsen impostor feelings in the long run, including avoiding situations that might trigger those feelings, overworking, or hiding failures out of shame and fear of judgement.

As you transition to the land of "grown-up" clinicians, now might be a good time to do an audit of your impostor-management strategies and adjust accordingly. Either you're going to need them, your colleagues are going to need them, or your clients will need them.

Licensure exams

Depending on where you are situated geographically and what type of clinician you are, you will likely have one or more licensing exams to complete post-graduation before you can practice independently. Among my fellow clinicians, I've seen all different approaches to preparing for licensing exams. I had one supervisor who decided to take the very-expensive Examination for the Professional Practice of Psychology (EPPP) without preparing at all, figuring that over 10 years of study in psychology should be plenty. I can't fault that logic in theory but in practice, she failed and had to redo it (more importantly, she had to pay the eye-watering fees again). I had other friends who spent every waking minute that they weren't working studying, which is the more common strategy though it may at times be overkill.

Here's the deal: most of these exams are pass/fail and there is no value or benefit to aiming for an A+. Your state or provincial licensing body will tell you what marks you need to attain to pass and be eligible to use the professional title of your choice but there is absolutely no benefit whatsoever to putting in the extra effort required to ace the exams; it won't make you a better clinician (Sharpless & Barber, 2009). For example, the ethics exam I took required that I choose the best answer to a dilemma from amongst four reasonably correct answers, with the goal being to identify the absolute best action to take first. It's great that I was able to select the best choice in most of the scenarios, but in real life, I'd probably implement all four solutions, as well as consulting colleagues and possibly some other problem-solving too.

I'd like to tell you that I played it cool and put in just enough effort to clear the bar on my licensing exams but you can probably tell by now that I didn't. Take it from someone who wasted her time getting that A+ only to discover (1) clients don't care, (2) employers don't care, and (3) I could have been spending that time doing literally anything else and would have been happier (looking at cat pictures on the Internet, for example). Grit your teeth, get them done, and then high-five yourself because you are honestly, truly, finally, without-a-doubt done taking exams in your life! Unless that is you need to move to another state or province...

Practical strategies for big days

As you complete your training program, there may be a few Very Important Days (VIDs): defending your thesis, sitting for a licensing exam, or interviewing for an internship or a job are some possibilities. Here are a few practical thoughts:

- If you have the choice, plan around yourself. If you're going to fret all morning and work yourself into a complete state, don't schedule exams or defenses for the afternoon. If you struggle to get up early even when there's a lot at stake, strategize accordingly. Don't give yourself an extra hurdle to leap on an already-big day.

- Don't worry too much about sleep the night before your VID. If you got a decent sleep two nights before, you'll probably be okay running on nerves and adrenaline. That being said, you may crash immediately after your big event, so make sure you've left some nap time in your schedule before the celebrations you have planned. And maybe go easy on the coffee so as not to throw gasoline on what may already be a significant case of the jitters.
- Leave more time than you think you may need for dressing and grooming. Plan for ripped seams, coffee stains, lost buttons, missing shoes, uncooperative cowlicks, and other minor disasters that could distract you from the task at hand.
- Make a checklist for items you need to bring with you, either on your phone or, if you're the old-fashioned type, with pen and paper. Tissues, water bottle, snacks, spare memory key, speaking notes – whatever equipment you will need. Start this list a week in advance so that you have plenty of time to remember random items. I find meditation sessions almost always help me to remember things I've forgotten or need to do.
- Check for construction along planned travel routes. I promise you that, at least in Canada, construction crews and giant pits in the road will spring up overnight if you have somewhere to be at a certain time the next day. Also, research parking lots or relevant public transit information.
- Meals: I wish I had something helpful to contribute here but unfortunately, I have made the mistakes both of eating too much (upset stomach at my doctoral defense) and too little (loud rumbling halfway through the EPPP). I think the main takeaway here is to pack both snacks and over-the-counter stomach remedies.

Know that minor glitches are likely, if not certain, to happen but most will probably be quite manageable. My VIDs were marked by stomach issues, hair problems, wrong directions, late thesis committee members, and unexpectedly finding out that the ethics exam monitor was the supervisor who'd been training me for the past year, so he would literally be staring at me while I tried to answer questions correctly (no pressure!). I survived every last one of them (more or less) and you will too. Probably.

Becoming the authority figure, or is there an adultier adult available?

I was getting ready for an outpatient therapy appointment at my job in a hospital when a supervisee came to my door and said, "Dr. Ménard, can I talk to you?" I replied, "I have a client coming in five minutes, can this

wait?" The student, normally very quiet and soft spoken, was unexpectedly forceful in her response: "No!!" As it turns out, her judgement was
very accurate: a patient had expressed very clear homicidal intent towards
a specific person with a detailed plan and ready access to a weapon. More
importantly, this patient was about to be discharged. This was a crisis
situation that required us to pull in various other team members quickly
to coordinate a response that ultimately involved psychiatry, nursing, and
one unusually psychologically minded trauma surgeon.

In the years since then, I've had a lot of students knock on my door with
expressions of terror on their faces, and there's always a moment of panic
for me too when that happens. For a split-second, I'm convinced that the
student is going to have some kind of problem I've never seen before and
I'll have absolutely no idea what to do or where to start; presumably, we
will then both melt into one unified puddle of panic, and I'm not sure what
happens after that. So far this hasn't happened, but my mind persists in
telling me that the next one will certainly be THE BIG ONE. My mind is
very short on details about "THE BIG ONE" and what it might actually
look like other than "BIG" and "TERRIBLE" so I'd better get ready.

Often, my supervisees' feelings of panic are quite out of proportion to
the actual problem. For the last few years, I have taught a graduate-level
class in CBT where most of the students are seeing their very first clients
for intervention; invariably, at least one of my student clinicians will get
worried and upset if their client has any history of suicidal ideation, no
matter how long ago or how mild the thoughts (Kleespies et al., 1993).
This kind of situation usually just requires a thorough check-in with the
student about whether they did a detailed risk assessment with the client,
and then we're good to go after a few minutes of deep breaths and reassur-
ances that they handled the situation correctly. Sometimes the anxiety is
occasioned by a bigger problem but one that is ultimately manageable; for
example, paperwork that fell through the cracks or a client showing symptoms that are quite different from their initial presentation and that might
require a shift in the treatment plan. And sometimes, like the example we
started with, there really is a genuine crisis to manage; however, in those
moments, it's always great to model seeking consultation from others. For
the supervisee, there can be something very validating in seeing that the
problem that was so concerning to them is of sufficient size and complexity
to require a team to solve it. And, frankly, no one really operates alone in
this field: reaching out to others is how I respond to my own clinical crises
and it's worked.

So far, I've always managed to provide sufficient adulting despite my
nagging suspicion that another adult would probably adult better than
I did. I am very curious to know if anyone ever completely settles into

the role of "authority figure" or if we all just keep looking for the "Head Adult" until the day we retire. I suspect it's the latter.

Clinical stamina

When you first start training, you might find yourself feeling wiped out by just one session – researching disorders and reading up on interventions, preparing for the therapy hour, getting through the session itself, completing any necessary notes or other administrative paperwork, watching the video or listening to the audio, and attending supervision. Initially, it's a lot, and you might yourself feeling very daunted at the idea of managing a full schedule of clients down the road.

This concern is entirely normal and valid. Please know that as you "grow up" clinically, some tasks will take less energy and you will also become more efficient. Once you've written a few dozen session notes, you will become faster and more efficient in producing them. Once you've seen a handful of clients, you'll need less energy in session to make sure that you're simultaneously taking notes, building the alliance, and staying on track of time. Over time, you'll see fewer brand-new problems that require a dive into the literature. In the meantime, be patient with yourself as you build your strength and stamina.

Keep in mind also that everyone has types of presenting problems that are more challenging for them than others, and this may continue throughout your professional life. Some clinicians like working with clients who have personality disorders, but others find these symptoms overwhelming and exhausting. One colleague told me she planned to centre her career around clients with disordered eating but soon realized there was no way she could manage that full-time. I went to a job interview once with a private practice therapist who told me that she saw ten clients a day, every day, one session leading directly to the next. It was very unclear to me where she found time to do her paperwork, return phone calls, or even go to the bathroom, and it didn't seem appropriate to ask at a job interview. I have another clinician friend who has never seen more than three clients in a day because she knows herself and this is the limit of what she can do well.

Try, if you can, to make your schedule work for you. As a student, you may not be in complete control of your calendar but if you have any flexibility, organize your days based not only on the total hours you have to put in but also on the types of activities you need to do. If you have a client with complex presenting problems, a new client or a meeting with a demanding supervisor, don't stack your day with other challenges. Plan your one really difficult activity and then use the rest of the day for less-demanding tasks – clients with more straightforward presenting prob-lems, watching therapy tapes or other administrative activities. "Getting it all over with" seems like a great idea until you're in the middle of that day and you wonder what jackass signed you up for this nightmare (in my case, it's almost always past Dana, who has a wildly inaccurate under-standing of what future Dana will be able to manage). You will ultimately figure out your sweet spot for the amount and type of work as an inde-pendent clinician.

Taking time to breathe between transitions

I finished my internship on a Friday in August. My husband made me a nice dinner on Saturday, I went to the beach with a friend on Sunday, and then I jumped straight into full-time work on the Monday. Please, go ahead and judge me for this behaviour; to this day, I cannot adequately explain why I didn't take a few days or even a few weeks to breathe after finishing 12 years total of university education.

Before you jump into the real world, take a breather of some kind. I understand that a lot of people may not have the finances to take a sig-nificant amount of time off, but please do what you can. Have a party with friends, have a quiet get-together with family, go away for the weekend with your partner, go on a silent retreat by yourself, have a big bonfire of all the stupid papers you've ever had to write. Mark the end of this chapter in whatever way makes the most sense to you but take the time to mark it. Life moves pretty fast. If you don't stop and look around once in a while – wait, I think I might have stolen this. The point is, you need to stop and celebrate yourself, to mark the end of all that training and grind-ing and suffering. You've achieved something momentous, something you were only dreaming of many years ago. Give it a minute to sink in.

Conclusion

I'm sure you've heard of the 90/10 rule: 90% of a project will take 10% of your time and the last 10% of a project will take 90% of your time. This is very applicable to graduate training programs in mental health, but in this case it's less so about time and more about energy and motivation. The last 10% of your program is likely to be where some of the biggest chal-lenges lie like exams and internships and dissertations defenses. Take heart that your training will end someday and some of the situations currently making your life very challenging will just be funny anecdotes you tell at a party years down the line. Or you'll have to write a book to process the trauma, like me and my internship applications. Either way, you'll survive.

Chapter 5

Self-care

Ah, self-care – no topic more clearly illustrates the embarrassing disconnect between what we mental health professionals preach to clients and what we practice ourselves. Many of us spend our academic years leaping from one deadline to the next, one class to the next, one item on our to-do list to the next. We usually aren't taught how to practice adequate self-care in our training programs but are instead given seemingly contradictory directives from our teachers: "Take care of yourself so you can take care of your clients!" but also "Write eight session notes, finish five reports, and mark 200 midterms in the next week." It's no wonder we struggle to find an appropriate work–life balance post-graduation.

I am no exception to the above description. I will freely admit that most of the writing for this chapter took place while I was (1) teaching a full course load, (2) leading multiple large research projects, and (3) figuring out how to parent a toddler – all of these were challenging, messy endeavours but in very different ways. Let's be clear right from the start that I'm just as flawed as everyone else in this field and part of my motivation for creating this chapter was to serve as a very long reminder to myself. However, my main motivation is that I want better things for the next generation of mental health professionals because I believe that one of the most important steps we need to take is to normalize the prioritization of self-care. This chapter may be a little more directive (okay, bossier) than other chapters, but I promise it's for your own good. Please understand that I'm not trying to give you something else to feel guilty about – I'm trying to give you the permission you need to put this at the top of your to-do list, and to push back on the forces that would interfere with this.

Self-care isn't a bonus – it's mandatory

If you remember just one idea from this chapter, let it be this: self-care is not optional. It's not like cleaning your baseboards or making your own almond milk or flossing your teeth (with apologies to my dentist). It is not

DOI: 10.4324/9781003355366-7

something you do if you have enough time left over after you've done the other *much more* important things. Self-care needs to be part of your routine, built into the framework of your day-to-day life and, most importantly, non-negotiable, no matter what else is happening because there will *always* be other stuff that's happening.

It's also not something you do once you notice that you need to do it: by the time you are feeling tired all the time, getting irritable with everyone, and over-indulging in unhealthy coping strategies (e.g., alcohol, substances, unsettling amounts of reality television), the situation has already gone too far. The time you need to refuel your fuel tank is when it is half-empty, not when the indicator is on red and your car starts to make an obnoxious pinging noise. True story: at one unusually busy point in my career, I had a dream that I was driving a car with a dark sticker covering up the fuel gauge so that I couldn't see how much gas I had left. The sticker then slowly peeled away to show that the tank was empty and I was running on fumes. I include this story as an illustration that (1) even people who should know better can let self-care slide and (2) you don't always need deep psychoanalysis to understand your dreams.

In therapy, you are your own tool – wait, that sounds weird. What I mean to say is that people in every other profession have instruments that they require to do their jobs, and part of their work involves caring for those instruments so that they can do their jobs properly. A chef sharpens their favourite knives, a barista cleans the espresso machine, a physician checks if their stethoscope is...on? I don't know anything about stethoscopes. The point here is that it's certainly nice to have a clipboard and a comfortable chair and maybe a plant in the corner of your office, but none of those things are truly mandatory. The only thing that is mandatory for therapy is you, so you need to take care of you to make sure that you are the most effective you available. Your clients deserve your very best work and so do you.

I'll say it again for those in the cheap seats at the back: self-care is not optional, and it will continue to be non-optional all the way through your career so get into the habit early and practice it with unrelenting dedication. Make sure you've got your stethoscope on so you can be the best therapist you can be.

Is this a self-care issue or a systems issue?

Before we go any further into the question of self-care, let's pause and consider whether the "self" part is even relevant to the situation causing you to need care. When it comes to work-induced stress, please, please always let your first question be, "Is this a 'me' problem or a 'systems' problem?" It's very important that you don't confuse the two, as both the contributors to the problem and the remedies for it are very different. Here are some handy diagnostic questions: does your workplace inevitably drive almost everyone there bananas? Is there high turnover and rampant cynicism amongst nearly all the employees? Do people smirk when you tell them where you work and say, "So how's *that* going?" These are all good indicators of systems issues that characterize toxic workplaces and contribute to burnout in employees (Moss, 2019). Have a look also at this handy table:

A "you" thing	A systems thing
You schedule more than your ideal number of clients per day because you can't stand disappointing anyone	Your workplace expects you to carry a caseload in excess of your own self-assessed capacity
You lack experience with a client group or problem	Your workplace does not support you in developing the necessary competencies and skills to work with the population you serve
Everyone is irritating you today	Everyone is irritating everyone all the time
You sometimes have trouble getting out of bed in the morning	Regular tears in your car before you walk into work

Here's another diagnostic I've found accurate across different settings: do people at your workplace take lunch breaks and, if so, do they take them with each other? Substitute "lunch breaks" for "short walks," "casual chats," "coffee," or "post-work get togethers" but the point remains – I've never worked in a toxic setting where anyone wanted to spend any extra time with one another, whereas short connections with colleagues usually happened daily at healthy workplaces.

Unfortunately, the remedies for systems issues are often not in your hands, and fighting for change in this type of situation can be long, slow, difficult, and painful. Only you can decide if other compensating factors at that site (e.g., salary, benefits, health insurance) make it worth staying. You might decide that in the interests of your sanity, you'll stay in the job for now, keep your head down, and not address any of the issues yourself. You might choose one problem on which to spend your time and energy, or you might decide to be a one-person revolutionary and fight the system every chance you get. Keep in mind that the solution you implement in one time period ("Deal with all the things!!") doesn't have to be the one you employ down the road ("Deal with just this one thing!!" or "Get the hell out of this place!").

For your ongoing health and wellbeing, it's important that you don't mistake systems issues for your own problems. You absolutely, positively can't self-care your way into making peace with a toxic workplace: no amount of yoga or mindful breathing will make up for feeling regularly disrespected and undervalued, and don't let anyone try to convince you otherwise. Employee "wellness" emails, I'm looking at you.

Set your limits and stick to them

Some of the best advice I ever got about graduate school came from a senior graduate student when I was preparing to enroll, who said, "Treat it like a job: don't work evenings, weekends, or holidays." The clearly missing caveat here was "extremely low-paying job," but the rest of the statement was true. With a few exceptions, I followed that dictum throughout grad school and it allowed me to get my work done efficiently while also being a reasonably happy person, or as happy as one can be upon entering grade 22, as my grandmother once referred to it. My fellow graduate students, many of whom seemed to work 24/7/365, were not especially happy and none of them completed the program any faster than I did, including the classmate who insisted that her boyfriend drive in complete silence for 16 hours on the way to and from a vacation so that she could focus on schoolwork in the car and the student, who upon hearing that I intended to graduate in six years, snarked "I guess you're not going to publish much."

Boundaries are the *sine qua non* of self-care – it doesn't really matter what you do for self-care as long as you have the time and energy to do it, which you will only get if you set boundaries. Establishing and maintaining boundaries will also enable you to be a better role model for your clients, colleagues, and supervisees.

How do you know what your limits should be? Excellent question, dear reader. I invite you to consider that beloved strategy that you've probably already discussed in one of your intervention courses: tracking. For a week or two, note down when you started work, when you stopped, what you did, and, most importantly, how you felt in your mind, body, and spirit. This will give you some valuable data to better understand the connection between your workload and your wellbeing, as well as a starting point for making some changes if they are needed. If you're feeling burned out and overwhelmed, try dialing some or all of your activities back by 10% and then re-evaluate in a few weeks. You might also consider keeping up with this tracking as a self-care intervention in and of itself: a friend of mine keeps a tally of what she's agreed to do on a weekly, monthly, and annual basis and sets limits for certain activities. For example, once she has signed up to do three guest lectures for the semester, she's done and can't accept any more invitations of this type until the following semester.

In terms of practicalities, boundaries should involve rules about the days you work and the hours you'll put in on those days. You should also have rules also about what "counts" as work; for example, writing clinical notes is definitely work but work-related reading may not be very taxing to you. Do not, *under any circumstances*, make an exception for email. And then when you hit your work limit just stop – don't check your email, don't open your calendar, just walk away from your electronic devices, or at least turn off your notifications. Set work aside until work hours start again. Did you feel uncomfortable just reading those sentences? That may be a good sign this chapter is especially important for you, and you should probably go grab a highlighter to reinforce key messages (paper copies only).

Here is the big secret to work–life balance: you can't wait for work to cooperate. It might be tempting to say that you'll implement some tough boundaries as soon as the next big thing wraps up, whether that's a training placement, a set of applications, an important thesis document or whatever else is currently giving you conniptions. But life isn't going to cooperate and give you a relatively chill stretch of several weeks so that you can finally just get your stuff together once and for all. I know because I've been waiting for my chill stretch for the last 20 years or so, and it just doesn't seem to be coming. You need to set your boundaries first and then work backwards to determine how you'll get the work done within those constraints.

Communicating your limits with others

Now, I understand that setting boundaries is much easier said than done, particularly when you feel your standing in the academic power hierarchy is relatively low. Academia and the clinical world beyond are rife with people who will advocate taking time off and then call you at 9:30pm on a Saturday night to edit a journal article, insist that you mark final exams on December 24, or email to request you edit a report while in labour (sadly, all true examples). Often, your professors will extol the virtues of work–life balance while simultaneously heaping demands on you like cardigan-wearing dump trucks.

Keep in mind always that "No" is a complete answer. Don't be tempted to provide explanations or justifications; for example, don't say "No, I can't help because I'm not familiar with that project" because the message you're really sending at that point is "I really would like to do this thing you're asking of me, just help me problem-solve the barrier I just articulated." At that point, the other person has nothing to lose by chipping away at your explanation like a stubborn woodpecker – please feel free to visualize your supervisor or colleague as a stubborn woodpecker if it helps you to push back. Practice the following reply: "I can't take on (opportunity/task/imposition) but you can check back with me at (later date) or maybe reach out to (some other poor sucker)." Rehearse it with friends so that when you really need to say that sentence, it rolls fluently off your tongue.

Another strategy to reinforce the boundaries you set is to bring in the values that you know that person holds for your work; this perfectly legitimate and fair strategy effectively traps them in their own net. For example, "I know it's very important to you that I be an ethical clinician and that I get my paperwork done in a timely fashion, so with that in mind, I would not be able to take on another assessment at this time." Once you've made the connection between their request and the overall principles guiding the work, they will find it much harder to argue with your limit.

Another consideration, though this should *not* be your primary motivator, is the potential impact of allowing your limits to be violated on the limits set by other people. If there is some kind of formal boundary or rule about work (e.g., no more than 10 hours work per week as a teaching assistant) but you say yes to a violation, the requestor has now been reinforced for their bad behaviour and will likely continue to press others to break rules that were in place for the protection of the group overall. If you can't say no to protect yourself, say no to protect others in your group or who may be impacted in the future.

Setting limits with others will certainly feel uncomfortable at first if you are used to overworking and you might disappoint some people but just like every other challenge in life, it will feel easier and more natural over time. You will all get used to the new limits, I promise, and if other people remain cranky, at least you'll be well-rested and more prepared to deal with their BS.

Managing boundary-induced guilt

If you embody the self-sacrifice schema that is typical of many clinicians, i.e., everyone else's needs come first, then yours, your mind is likely to push back on setting work-related limits. Here are some potential objections and a matching set of handy reframes.

"The more time I spend learning, the better clinician I'll be! I just need to do more, more, more!" → You need time to effectively digest and consolidate your learning. You'll also have better attention and memory for your learning if you are rested.

"I just need to push through to get this work done, then I can take a break" → You could work 24 hours a day, 7 days a week and still not get it all done. Lean in to that discomfort. Taking breaks will push you to be more efficient in your working hours.

"My clients need me!" → Your clients need a well-rested, calm therapist, not someone who is so frazzled and overwhelmed they can't focus during session.

"But this is a really valuable learning opportunity, I really think I should sign up for this class/workshop/extra training." → Opportunities come back around. You won't get what you want out of it if you are drained.

You will almost certainly be tempted at some point to cancel your planned leisure in favour of (1) more work or (2) mindless leisure (e.g., Netflix and phone). Don't. Trips to the gym, doctor's appointments, visits with hard-of-hearing grandparents who refuse to wear their hearing aids – all of these activities take energy and may be at least somewhat challenging, but all of them will yield dividends to your future wellbeing. Consider what you'd tell a client under similar circumstances and then apply that wise advice to your hypocritical ass.

How to self-care

There's been a lot of money made in the so-called "wellness" industry over the last couple of decades – over $5.6 trillion, in fact (Global Wellness Institute, 2023) – but I promise you that real self-care is generally a lot cheaper than Gwyneth Paltrow would have you believe (Caulfield, 2015). If someone is advocating for a fancy, expensive new approach to looking after yourself, don't fall for the hype, in much the same way that you shouldn't buy "new therapy" hype. The boring "apples and oranges" of self-care are just as effective, if not more so, than the expensive options; for example, free yoga classes on YouTube do a lot of what a $25 class does and you can practice at home in your underwear without judgment.

I've noticed that a lot of the pushback around self-care from both clients and colleagues seems to stem from the view that self-care is defined by activities like getting a massage, taking a bath, or painting one's toenails. Certainly, if you enjoy these types of activities, dig in. I, myself, am very fond of a nail polish colour known as "Lost without my GPS", which is both (1) fetching and (2) accurate. But broaden your mind to include all kinds of activities that leave you feeling cared for and refreshed in all domains of your existence. Self-care can look like taking care of your body by eating right, getting enough sleep, exercising, keeping alcohol/drugs/tobacco to a minimum, and managing chronic medical issues. For example, making (and then keeping!) an appointment with your physio-therapist to follow up on nagging pain is self-care. Self-care can look like taking care of your space by paying your bills on time, calling a plumber before that clog threatens to flood your kitchen, or buying a furry blanket so that your therapy chair is as cozy as possible. Self-care can involve nurturing your relationships by taking a minute to text your dad a funny meme, watching a cheesy movie with your partner or joining a barber-shop chorus, if that happens to be your cup of tea. Self-care may include attending to your spiritual side by going to a service in your faith group or finding other ways to connect with something bigger than the day-to-day mundanities. Consider making self-care a group activity with other clinicians: take a weekly yoga class or karaoke night or maybe start some kind of fight club. Be creative, be expansive, be generous with your self-care but, most importantly, be consistent.

Pee first, then session notes

As you navigate your workdays, make sure that you take care of your basic biological needs: go to the bathroom, eat, add an extra layer if you're cold, take some pain medication if you have a headache. You wouldn't think I'd need to spell this out, but I've fallen into this trap more than once myself. Eating was a particular issue when I worked at a private practice and saw clients from 12 to 8pm. Being the good clinician that I was, I always tried to finish my session notes before I left the office for the day; however, rather than stop and take a few minutes to refuel, I'd try to power through the writing with my sad, depleted brain so that I could get home. Predictably, this approach was both (1) slow and (2) ineffective. It took more total time to get the notes done than it would have if I had taken a short break to stretch, eat something, or just get some fresh air, then written the notes.

Look after your body first and foremost. If you are physically uncomfortable in any way and there's something you can do about that, do that thing! Don't put off caring for your body by saying: "I'll just finish this session note, I'll just return this phone call, I'll just draft this email..." I promise, you will be a less-efficient, less-happy clinician if you do this routinely. If you struggle to pick on these cues within yourself until it's too late, make noticing these signs your first priority; for example, learn to eat when you're peckish rather than wait until you're ravenous. Practice noticing whispers before they become shouts.

To reinforce healthy behaviour in myself, I turned it into a bit of a mantra: "Eat first." I urge you to do this yourself – pick a self-care behaviour that you struggle to prioritize and turn it into a short, pithy phrase you can repeat to yourself as needed. Consider tattooing it on the inside of your arm as a reminder (unless it's "pee first", that might be a little weird).

Keeping work at work

The ability to compartmentalize – keeping thoughts and feelings about work at work – is critical for therapists' mental health (Posluns & Gall, 2020; Ziede & Norcross, 2020). It's the fundamental skill that will allow you to take evenings, weekends, and holidays off without spending the whole time ruminating about clients' progress or feeling guilty that you're taking time off at all. Here are some practical recommendations for how to compartmentalize:

- Apply what you're learning to yourself, whether it's thought records, mindfulness strategies, cognitive defusion, a two-chair exercise – anything that will target your guilty thoughts, worries, or rumination. At the very least, you'll understand better what you're asking of your clients and at best, the strategies that other clinicians have been recommending and practicing for decades might actually work.
- Always remember what your role is – to be a "good enough" therapist, not the most perfect therapist in the world. Being a perfect therapist is just plain impossible and even if it was, your clients would still retain their right to ignore your wisdom. Consider getting a bracelet made with the letters "WWAGETD?" – What Would A Good-Enough Therapist Do?
- Have a ritual to wrap up your workday. Finish your notes, tidy your space, clean your hot-beverage mug, make your to-do list for tomorrow, play an "end of work song" (I suggest "9 to 5" by our queen, Dolly Parton). The repetition of this habit over time will gradually condition your mind to the idea that you are about to leave work, and your work worries will stay at work until you return. Similarly, have another ritual when you arrive home. Go for a walk, take a shower, do some deep-breathing, or debrief with your partner, a roommate or a family member. Dogs are excellent listeners if ear scritches are involved. This second ritual will help signal to your mind that you are home now, and the main concerns should be "What shall we have for dinner?" and "Why is the dryer making a squeaky noise?", not "Why isn't my 4pm Thursday client making progress?"
- Make sure your off-hours are full of meaningful, life-affirming activities. Spend time with friends, do your hobbies, travel, exercise – whatever activities make you "you." Practice guitar, bake, read, rock-climb, or whatever else you do that reminds you that you're not *just* a therapist, you're a rock-climbing therapist.
- When you are genuinely concerned about a client's lack of progress or the severity of their issues and you find yourself frequently worrying about them outside of work, seek out supervision or consultation with

other clinicians. Get their opinion on the work you've done and make any changes that seem like a reasonable fit, keeping in mind also that the answer may be that you are doing as much as any reasonable clinician would do. If you've already graduated, consider joining a peer supervision group so that you have people in your life readily available for these moments.

Avoid academic martyrs

Any academic program that requires high marks and a boatload of extra-curriculars just to be admitted is bound to attract some real type-A personalities, some of whom may enjoy games of competitive martyrship. You may have already met some. If you've got three books to read, they've got seven; if you've got a 20-page paper to write, they have a 30-page paper; if you have 100 midterms to mark, they have 200. If you mention a new show that you're enjoying, they'll sigh and say they wish they had time to do such things but alas, they do not. They haven't been to the gym in six months, and they envy you the time you find to shower.

First of all, gross!! Showering is mandatory, people – we live in a society. Second of all, don't buy this nonsense! Pay close attention and you'll spot the inconsistencies in their behaviour; yes, they don't enjoy the same leisure activities as you, but they likely have their own that they're forgetting or downplaying. The student who would like to head home at 5pm but alas has too much paperwork is on social media every time you glance over at their screen. The person who wishes they could go to the gym like you do but is sadly unable due to their caseload has an updated manicure every week. Your classmate who can't find time to pick up a book for fun is nevertheless up-to-date on all the latest relationship drama of their favourite reality television stars. Don't let people make you believe that they do nothing but work and sleep, and don't let them shame you for your preferred leisure strategies. I promise, no one you know is actually a clinical robot, working effectively for 16 hours a day before powering down to recharge those empathy cells at night.

In my experience, it's best not to confront these people. Just nod empathically and skip off home to walk your dog, secure in the knowledge that taking the time to do this is making you a better therapist in the long run. Or at least a better dog parent, which is always worth doing.

Rough days

Alas, these are inevitable even for the best boundary-setting, self-care-practicing clinicians out there. A parking ticket, an argument with a partner, a cat who threw up on your bed at 5:20am – any and all of life's bullshit. I suspect it may be easier to hide a crotchety state of mind in other jobs (truck driver, for example, or lighthouse operator), but as a psychotherapist, your clients are going to expect a certain level of serenity from you, so here's how to fake that.

- Do the bare minimum. Obviously, you'll see your clients and write your notes but put off for another day what can wait: report-writing, annoying phone calls, complex emails, non-urgent tasks of any type.
- Do not *under any circumstances* attempt to take on activities that are aggravating to you on a good day. This may include meetings with colleagues you find frustrating, scoring tricky assessment measures, calls to insurance companies, or anything that requires deep breathing before you even start.
- Try to reset. Go for a 5-minute walk, phone someone you love, watch a funny video on YouTube, listen to your favorite song – anything to get your mind out of repeating its "anger mantra" over and over. Repeat as needed throughout the day. Make sure you compile this list of reset activities before you need it and put it somewhere obvious. You don't want to be trying to come up with ideas for peaceful, calming activities when you're ready to Hulk out.
- Lean into the work and let the clinical hour help you too. I've often found that really immersing myself in my clients' worlds gives me some much-needed perspective and distance from my own issues, or at least a 50-minute break.

Despite your best efforts, your clients may pick up on your mood, and you certainly don't want to gaslight them by pretending everything is fine when it isn't; however, you also don't want your clients to feel that they are now in the position of having to look after you. For these situations, I have some stock phrases handy for responding to expressions of concern: "I'm doing my best. How are you?" or "Today's a little rough but I'm managing." It's okay to be human; in fact, it's good to model that times can be tough for everyone, even therapists.

Rough days are inevitable, or at least they will be until boyfriends and cats get their respective acts together and just behave, but with a little readjusting, you can get through them. You will then be free to go home and become one with your sofa while you binge-watch reality TV until your brain melts – you've earned it!

How sick is too sick to work?

Like many type-A personalities, I struggle with taking time off. I have repeatedly pushed myself to keep working when it was painfully obvious that I should not have been. Case in point: I completed my final licensing exam while battling a lingering case of strep throat (ironically, it was the oral exam). Looking back, I can say that there are many days that I regret going in to work, and none at all where I regret staying home.

I strongly recommend that you tackle the question "How sick is too sick to work?" and identify your limits *before* you get sick. "Of course I wouldn't go in if I had a cold! What an absurd suggestion!" you might say to yourself. However, the morning you wake up with a headache or a scratchy throat or an upset stomach, it will be easy to rationalize going in. Cancelling an appointment with an abstract client is very easy, but cancelling on someone who you know is struggling and could use your support is very hard. This is why you need to create your rules for taking sick days before you need them. Sample rules might include "I don't go in to work for at least 24 hours after vomiting" or "I will wait until day five minimum of a cold to return", or "I can work with a headache but never a migraine." If you are feeling well enough to focus on your clients but are concerned about spreading a bug, doing sessions through teletherapy may be a compromise option (see Chapter 12).

The above recommendations refer to acute problems, but what if you have an ongoing, chronic issue that flares up and down, something that may leave you in significant pain or overwhelm you with fatigue like auto-immune conditions, fibromyalgia, or endometriosis? Chronic problems need a few more levels of planning as the disruptions are not just limited to your symptoms but also to specialist appointments required to manage the problem, and this scheduling may be outside of your control. During difficult times or prolonged episodes of illness, if you are in doubt of your clinical capacities, dial back. Remember: "Could have done more but didn't" is a different kind of mistake from "Overdid it and hurt someone/ myself" – most of us can probably live more easily with the first mistake compared to the second. As I recommended in Chapter 3, you'll need to share enough details about the situation with managers or supervisors to enable effective long-term planning. Explore with them how you can organize your clinical day around your periods of best functioning and titrate your workload based on your capacities, keeping in mind that the solution you implement during one season of life may need to be revisited should circumstances change. With clients, you'll need to be as transparent as you can about what changes might happen, how often they might happen, and what you will do to minimize the impact on them, while still ensuring that boundaries do not get blurred and clients shift their focus to your wellbeing.

If you are a caretaker for someone with an acute or chronic illness, you may have similar challenges (e.g., sudden session cancellations, reduced capacities for work at times). The above counsel applies: be proactive, be transparent, dial back as needed, and share as much as you feel comfortable with supervisors/managers and clients to plan effectively. When I took care of my father in the year leading up to his death, I sometimes had to have my phone on during sessions – usually a cardinal sin of psychotherapy – because I would have to arrange chemotherapy logistics or confirm scheduled CT scans. Every single client I worked with during this time was completely understanding. A few sessions were interrupted for short periods but we were always able to pick up the thread of the work and resume.

You are allowed, encouraged even, to be human, and human bodies tend to be fallible. You will be a better psychotherapist if you take care of your whole self, just as you would have your clients take care of theirs. Think of it as the Golden Rule of Psychotherapy – do unto yourself as you would have clients do unto themselves.

Conclusion

It's my dream someday that all clinical training programs will include a mandatory class called "Practice what we preach" with lectures about getting enough sleep and exercise, making time for socializing, finding time for spiritual connection, and, of course, lots and lots of homework focused on instilling healthy habits. Until that day comes, I think the most important thing we can do is model good self-care for our colleagues, our trainees, and our clients. I persist in believing it may be one of the most crucial determinants of the quality of our work as clinicians. We all deserve better, and that change starts with the care we take of ourselves.

Chapter 6

Professionalism

Is it okay to drink coffee in session? Can you wear jeans to work? What about cursing in session – always permissible, sometimes okay or never acceptable? These are all hot-topic and debatable issues under the wider umbrella of what constitutes "professional" behaviour for psychotherapists, and all of these choices have the potential to impact the therapeutic alliance with clients. Professionalism is an area where new trainees may feel particularly vulnerable: you are still in the process of developing your professional identity, behaviours considered appropriate in one setting may be deemed inappropriate in another, and errors in this domain can feel more consequential than other types of mistakes. Please rest assured that this chapter has no definitive answers whatsoever to any of these conundrums. Sorry! What we can do is talk it out and hopefully, you will find it easier to identify a set of choices that work for you.

Understanding professionalism

Defining, understanding, and embodying professionalism in our work is deeply cultural; "appropriate" therapeutic behaviour is likely to change across psychotherapeutic orientations, geographical locations, different professions, and time periods (Elizabeth & Callaghan, 2005; Hodges et al., 2019; McCluney et al., 2021). Professionalism will also depend on the demographics of the clinician and the client, and whether there are significant discrepancies between the two (e.g., old/young, male/female, racial minority/racial majority). However, the fluid nature of expectations for work-related behaviours does not exempt us from obeying those that apply to us here in North America in the early 21st century or, in other words, you don't get to curse like a sailor in session just because Australian therapists do (with apologies to my Aussie readers if I am wrong about this one).

I know we just spent a bunch of time on boundaries in the last chapter, but we're going to revisit the notion of boundaries here, in a slightly

DOI: 10.4324/9781003355366-8

different context. In the realm of professionalism, boundaries serve to protect the integrity of the relationships you have with your clients. Firm, professional boundaries help to remind your clients that you are not a friend, a surrogate parent, or a potential love interest (again, never *ever* sleep with your clients). You are a healthcare professional and the relationship you have with them, while intimate and at times intense, is going to reflect those limits. Your professional boundaries are communicated to your clients in every action you take: starting and ending sessions on time, keeping the session content focused on the client and their needs, dressing for the workplace, and returning emails and phone calls promptly. While I don't generally agree with clinicians who fall back on the "slippery slope" argument – one mildly problematic behaviour leads invariably to more grievous errors – I do think that a clinician wearing sweatpants to conduct a session is likely to cue an entirely different set of behaviours in a client than one wearing dress pants.

Here's a piece of blanket advice about how to be professional: if you are ever unsure about whether to relax a boundary, make the more conservative choice at first. You can always loosen up down the road, but you can rarely put the genie back in the bottle once it's out. Take it from someone who's made that mistake – I once disclosed my lack of religious beliefs to a client who was very insistent about having this information. The client then spent many subsequent sessions explaining to me that I would ultimately join them on the correct path (i.e., theirs) when my life became sufficiently challenging. Religious proselytizers at your front door are bad enough, but when they're sitting in the therapy room across from you, it can seriously derail the work you are meant to be doing.

Eating/drinking in session

Once upon a time, when I was in graduate school, a fellow student brought her travel mug into a session and sipped from it occasionally throughout the hour; as I recall, the client didn't comment on this behaviour. So why am I even sharing such an innocuous story you ask? Our clinical supervisor noticed this choice while reviewing my colleague's videotape of the session and we then spent 25 minutes in the next group supervision dissecting in detail the possible significance of the therapist's travel mug to the client. Did the client think she was distracted? Did the client feel the therapist was ungenerous for not offering a hot beverage to them? Did the client have concerns related to the content of the mug? What did the travel mug *mean* clinically? It was excruciating and we students talked about that supervision session for months. Many years later, I worked at a private practice that had an elaborate beverage cart conveniently stationed in the waiting room for the enjoyment of both clinicians and clients, featuring dozens of different hot beverages, including teas, coffees, and hot chocolate. At Christmas, we had a tureen of hot apple cider that was continually topped off by our dedicated administrative assistant; at major holidays, we had baskets of sugary treats available. The owner of that private practice believed as a matter of principle that clients who are physically comfortable and relaxed are more apt to open up and share difficult feelings and experiences; having seen the results, I agree with her approach.

If you've ever been in therapy yourself, take this moment to think back and ask yourself whether you ever noticed what your therapist was drinking in session. I'm willing to bet that unless they had a martini glass or a strong odour of gin coming from their mug, you didn't notice or care. This is my position: I don't think sipping from a beverage in session is a big deal and I don't think most clients have strong opinions on the issue.

I will acknowledge that questions about the role beverages may play in creating distraction during the session are fair: you don't want to be looking for your water glass when your client is finally disclosing a trauma that they've been holding in for years. However, I also think that distraction can go both ways. If you are physically uncomfortable in some way, you will probably struggle to focus on what your client is saying (see Chapter 5, p. 68). Most clients understand that as a human, you will occasionally have human needs, like thirst, and they are happy for you to take care of those needs so that you can focus on them. Until I see some data on the disruptive impact on clients of therapists managing dehydration, I will continue to have my water bottle readily available in session.

Food is another matter; personally, I have never eaten in session, but I have heard from other clinicians that they munched on a few crackers during the clinical hour because of health issues like low blood sugar or pregnancy. If you fall into this category, transparency will be your friend: you don't have to give clients all the details about your medical situation, but you should let them know that for health reasons, you might need a little snack to ensure your continued focus on them. Just make it crackers and not a tuna fish sandwich (too smelly) or a steak (too tricky to cut while balancing on your lap).

Touching your clients

I know I've told you several times now that you must never, ever sleep with your clients, which is always, under every possible circumstance Bad Touching. But let's stop for a minute and consider the possibility that there could be Good Touching in psychotherapy. This has been a deeply fraught issue in our field (Bonitz, 2008; Damon et al., 2022). Some mental health professionals are of the opinion that any kind of physical touch between a therapist and a client has the potential to become problematic over time;

on the other side, there are those who say that certain kinds of touching can be humanizing and occasionally necessary.

I definitely fall in the latter camp: some touching, now and then, with very specific clients, and for very clear reasons. The most common kind of touch I'm talking about here is a brief hug. Moments that have led to hugs in my career have included termination sessions – by far the most common time for a client to ask for a hug – and variations on "geez, that was an intense session," including disclosures of trauma or awful news of various kinds (e.g., unexpected deaths). My experience to date is that most clients understand that therapy does not routinely involve hugs or touch, and they also do not expect exceptions to be made routine. I've never had a client who asked for a hug after a tough session start asking for one on a weekly basis. Certainly, there are settings and populations where it is probably wise to have a "no touching at any time" policy, including certain forensic settings, clients with complex personality issues, and clients with histories of boundary violations (e.g., abuse survivors). When I did a placement in a prison, I worked with a client who wanted to put his hand on my back as we walked down the hallway – not a great choice with that patient population anyway but particularly not in a setting where many patients' hygiene was on the lax side.

If you personally are not comfortable with hugging or other forms of touch, feel free to say, "I'm sorry, there's a policy about not touching in this setting," even if there isn't one, which gets you off the hook without shaming your client for needing some human contact. You can then identify alternative strategies for creating a sense of connection, warmth, and groundedness for when those are particularly needed. Maybe some synchronized deep breathing or a discussion about a cuddly pet? If you are comfortable with a handshake, I have sometimes offered a "warm handshake," i.e., a two-handed shake where you cover the back of the client's shaking hand with your non-shaking hand. You might also consider a fist bump or a high-five, depending on the client population, but that's up to you as well. You'll definitely want to take the age of your client into account as older generations may require some explanation and practice to pull off the fist bump.

Therapist self-disclosure

It's a cliché but the psychotherapeutic relationship is very different from all other relationships, which includes relationships with other healthcare professionals. For example, I know that my massage therapist broke up with her last boyfriend because he sat around the house all day smoking pot and doing nothing (probably a good call). One of the nurses who looked after my daughter when she was born gained 80 lbs during her own pregnancy but her son weighed just 8 lbs at birth. My dentist has three kids and regularly daydreams about fixing all the damaged smiles he sees at the gym. In all of these cases, the other professional disclosed this information to me voluntarily and with little-to-no prompting; I will acknowledge that I have a very severe case of "Resting Talk-to-me Face,"[1] which probably contributes to the problem. In fact, everything I know about my dentist has been strictly one-way communication as I usually have a mouth full of instruments in these moments. Given the landscape of different approaches to disclosing personal information even amongst other health-care fields, it's not altogether surprising that clients don't understand why we may be reluctant to answer questions about our own personal lives.

There have been reams upon reams written about therapist self-disclosure (e.g., Hanson, 2005; Ziv-Beiman, 2013), ranging from "share almost nothing" to "sharing may be necessary for effective psychotherapy." Early in my training, I was told by supervisors, "If a client asks you a personal question, don't answer. Shoot the question right back to them automatically." So if the client asks if you have children, you say, "I'm curious why you're asking me that question." If a client asks where you're going on vacation, you say "I'm curious why that matters to you?" If they bring up a problem with their child and ask if you're a parent, you say, "I'm curious how that information will be helpful to you?" I think I understand now that these supervisors were just being cautious with a room full of beginning clinicians who had yet to develop a sense of professional judgement; however, as a blanket approach, I think this is a terrible idea. At its worst, this kind of dedication to complete opacity on the part of the clinician can rise to the level of gaslighting clients. I once knew a therapist who identified as gay, whose office was located in the city's gay district, who served a primarily gay clientele, and who had pride flags in his office, but who did not disclose his own sexual orientation. Similarly, if you wear a traditional wedding band on the traditional finger or you have a photo of your child on your desk, there is no point in deflecting questions about your marital or parental status; in any case, I think it would be even weirder to have a photo of a child on your desk if they weren't a relative.

When it comes to voluntary therapist self-disclosure, to my mind, clients are human and they care about you as a person; most questions of this type directed at clinicians are clients' ways of showing an interest, as we

---

1 "Resting Talk-to-me Face" is a little-known phenomenon that is the opposite of "Resting Bitch Face." It causes strangers to spill intimate personal details with very little provocation in various public settings like trains or physicians' waiting rooms. It is generally considered an asset in therapy-related professions but can be a liability for a therapist who just wants to mind their own business outside of work. I suggest big headphones and possibly a garlic-heavy lunch if you're going on a long flight.

generally do when we like people. Bidirectional caring is important for healthy, functional therapeutic alliances (Baier et al., 2020; Bowie et al., 2016; Littauer et al., 2005). I think questions about vacation destinations or whether you have pets or where you went to school are fair game to answer, if you feel comfortable disclosing this information. I will certainly admit to clients that I have dealt with universal human issues like anxiety, insomnia, or procrastination as a therapeutic tool. I have even shared information about personal losses when I thought a client would benefit from knowing that I have lived experience to better understand their situation (for example, loss of a parent or miscarriage).

Now and then, client questions may reflect poor boundaries or social skills. For example, "Don't you think my mother acted like a complete bitch?!" – definitely don't answer this one – or "Oh my God, how old are you?" in the first session with a brand-new client. Over time, your clinical spidey-sense will develop and you'll generally know the difference between an innocuous question, that you may choose to answer, and an inappropriate one, where you probably should pull the Uno reverse card. The main question you need to answer is why you are choosing to share some detail and what you hope to accomplish with sharing; your answer should reflect the client's needs, not yours. Likewise, know your "bailout point" for self-disclosure (Bray, 2019) – yes I have kids, yes these are their ages, no, I'm not going to tell you at what age they potty-trained (I presume my daughter will thank me when she's older).

Critiques of your professionalism

There's a lot of terminology out there that can be misused to criticize mental health professionals in training without being specific or constructive; unfortunately, I've seen the term "unprofessional" applied frequently in this context when the issue was actually a personal one, but the complainant wanted to disguise the nature of the problem for their own nefarious reasons. "You question our outdated practices in this clinic and we don't like that," is not something managers are allowed to say but, "Your behaviour in the workplace is unprofessional and we don't like that" has a nice vague ring to it and won't trigger an official internal review.

This may be a particular issue with clinicians who fall into minoritized or marginalized groups. "You're trans and that makes me uncomfortable," is not something a supervisor can say but can be hidden by, "You wear nail polish in sessions and that's unprofessional," while conveniently ignoring the fact that cis trainees are not forbidden from wearing nail polish. There is a long history of policing the hairstyles of Black professionals and many institutional settings will have policies in place solely to target afros and other natural hairstyles (Koval & Rosette, 2021; Opie & Phillips, 2015). I'm sure if you are a member of such a group, you've been dealing with this kind of nonsense for a long time, and you may not be surprised to see it happening in therapeutic settings. I want to believe that issues related to equity, diversity, inclusion, and justice (EDIJ) are trending in the right direction within the mental health space, that there's more awareness of how the "phobias" and the "isms" are built right into our definitions of "professional," but I also know there's a lot of work still to be done. If you fall into a category where there's the potential for comments about your professionalism to be informed by prejudice, may I recommend that you find a mentor who falls into the same group and who will serve as someone with whom to process these types of comments. It could be someone you know in person, someone you've worked with in the past or someone you connect with in an online group – it just has to be someone you can trust, who can tell you whether another supervisor has a point and there's a change you need to make or whether they are just being a racist/homophobic/transphobic/sexist/ableist asshat.

Being told that your behaviour or presentation is unprofessional is usually difficult to hear. Certainly, I would advise you to ask for clarification and examples of the type of problematic behaviour under question, but if the comment is intended as a cover-up for more personal agendas, you may not get any, or you might get less-than-useful feedback. You may consider switching supervisors if possible or, depending on the severity and frequency of such comments, another training site. I urge you to report this information to the powers-that-be in your program so that they can establish whether the site/supervisor has a track record of this sort of behaviour and hopefully save another trainee from enduring similar nonsense.

What to wear

Consistent with the fuzzy guidelines that characterize a lot of the "professionalism" discourse, dress codes governing appropriate workplace apparel for therapists are often unclear, and usually more notable for their prohibitions than their recommendations. "Nothing too high, too low, or too tight" is how the expectations were communicated to me in one setting but who sets the bar on high, low, or tight? Do we measure the depth of the plunge or the length of a skirt in inches? Should it also depend on your body type, which can drastically affect fit? Not long after that unhelpful recommendation, I took a dress to a tailor to remedy a neckline that was too low for my taste and jokingly asked the elderly Middle Eastern owner if he could "unsexy" it for me, to which he replied, with a completely straight face, "'Sexy' is in the eye of beholder." Indeed!

Dress codes in clinical settings are primarily created to guide clients in perceiving us a certain way – as healthcare professionals – but the reality is that we can stack the deck as much as possible but we still won't have total control over how we are perceived. For example, when I worked at a prison, I exclusively wore loose clothing that covered me from neck to wrists to ankles, and I still got inappropriate sexual comments weekly. In that case, the issue was largely one of context: I was a new, young female person in a setting where the male/female ratio was 90:10 and new people showed up only rarely. Most of the patients were probably (1) very bored and (2) quite horny. This was the same setting where a nurse told me I shouldn't wear drapey scarves as these constituted a strangulation risk should a client become annoyed with me. This very helpful advice was shared with me 11 months into a 12-month placement, but I am happy to report that no strangulation attempts had been made prior to receiving that advice. So some dress code rules were created for your protection and you should definitely adhere to those wherever relevant (see also: wearing open-toed shoes in settings where people might vomit on you).

Some general guidelines on dress may still be useful. Certainly, you wouldn't want to wear the same outfits to see clients as you would to watch Netflix, hang out with your friends, or bar hop; you should be thinking more along the lines of dressing for a job interview or meeting your significant other's parents for the first time. You want the client to look at you and think that your relationship will be professional; you will not be bingeing content together, hanging out, or getting jiggy with it, in any sense of the word "jiggy." Depending on the age bracket of your clientele, you might want to dress in certain ways to connect with them; for example, if you often work with teenagers, you might want to avoid clothes that project the appearance of being stuffy or out-of-touch (e.g., ties, pants with creases). When I worked at one busy hospital, we were required to wear white coats on the patient floors for infection control, but I made a point of leaving mine unbuttoned enough so that patients and their families could see that I was not wearing scrubs underneath. Anyone who has spent any time in a hospital knows that people wearing scrubs are prone to dashing around and rarely have time to chat. I wanted to subtly show patients and their families that I was different kind of white coat and would have time to sit and talk with them about their concerns.

Your clothes don't just help put clients in the right mindframe, they can also help you get your head in the game. When I first started as a therapist, I was terrified going into most of my sessions. It felt like there were a million things to keep track of and so many decisions to be made, so many different ways to get things wrong. Clothes helped project an aura of confidence that I just didn't feel yet due to rampant impostor feelings (see

Chapter 4, p. 54). "Look at my blazer," I imagined saying to clients. "Only a real therapist would wear a blazer so I must know what I'm doing. Don't even get me started on these loafers."

Bottom line: there's no universal agreement on what constitutes "professional dress." An outfit deemed "inappropriate" in one setting might be considered entirely appropriate and even "cute" in another. You might choose to dress a certain way to give yourself a boost or to connect with clients. Definitely keep safety in mind, whatever that means in your setting, and know deep in your heart that " 'Sexy' is in the eye of the beholder."

Social media

This is how old I am: I started graduate school before Twitter and Instagram even existed. Facebook was around, but site membership was still restricted to post-secondary students and not the ubiquitous, everyone-and-their-grandma space it is now. Blogs were quite popular but not easy to find unless you were looking for one specifically, so it was very unlikely that clients would accidentally stumble upon them. I think it's safe to say that my professors had no idea what kind of landscape we would eventually be navigating as mature clinicians.

It's fair to be concerned about what clients might learn about you from your Internet presence and how that might affect the therapeutic relationship, and I've seen a variety of approaches to this issue by myself and other clinicians. Many simply crank up the privacy settings on all their social media accounts and live with the problem of family and friends having trouble finding them; some see this as a feature, not a bug. Some use a fake name, usually some variation on their real names (e.g., First name + last initial), while others maintain separate accounts for their personal and professional lives. Some people just don't have any social media accounts: these are the most productive people of all.

Either way, you may find yourself navigating friend/follow requests to your personal accounts from clients on various platforms. Unless your posts are exclusively mental-health themed, you should probably turn down these requests and address it in the next session. You can use some variation on: "I noticed you sent me this request but I turned you down. Our relationship needs to focus on you and your needs." I suspect this problem may be a generational issue that will dissipate over time. Older users of social media may be less likely to understand the implicit rules governing its use compared to younger users, much like how people over a certain age need to be reminded to silence their phones in theatres while the younger generation has literally never taken their phone off silent.

Expect the unexpected

The setting for this little melodrama was a private practice job I had recently started; more specifically, I worked in a basement office featuring a well-style window. I had only been there for a few months and was still in that honeymoon phase where I was trying to impress upon my boss that I was truly the best, most professional choice she could have made. I was in a session with a client when they remarked out-of-the-blue, "Is that a squirrel in your window?" I looked up, caught a glimpse of fur, and said, "Yeah, probably. It'll find its way out." The session continued, uneventfully. As I was writing up the note, immediately afterwards like a good therapist, I looked up and beheld not a squirrel as my client thought but a possum! It was a baby possum that had become stuck in my window well and couldn't climb up the corrugated metal to get out. Even though it was on the other side of the window, this is likely the closest I've ever been to such an animal. It's important to note also that I'm a city girl and what I know about critter-wrangling is very minimal. So I did what any self-possessed, over-educated, reasonable 31-year old would do: I called my dad, in a city 800 kilometers away. The call wasn't recorded but here's my recollection of it:

Me: Dad! Dad! Dad! There's a possum in my office window! A possum!!! What do I do??
My dad: A possum in your office?
Me: No, in my window well! It's stuck and it can't get out!
My dad: Have you called animal control?
Me: Yes, but it's been 30 minutes and they're not here.
My dad: Well, I'm sure they've got lots of possums to rescue, they'll get to you eventually.
Me: Should I tell my boss? She's in a session but maybe she'd want to know that the animal control people are coming.
My dad: No, you're a big girl, you can handle this.

Readers, I did not feel like a "big girl" in this moment. The rest of the afternoon's sessions were challenging as I attempted to focus on the clients' concerns while not swiveling my head around every few minutes to check on the possum or straining to listen for the arrival of animal control. Anyways, fully two hours later, the animal control guy finally arrived with a very sophisticated instrument he called a "grabber," hoisted the possum out of the window well by the armpits, and dumped it in our parking lot, whereupon the possum waddled off, no doubt to tell his friends about the exciting afternoon he'd had. By the time I was able to update my boss on the situation, it had been effectively managed and she approved my course of action, as well as the decision not to disturb her. The only lasting outcome was that the practice secretary used a picture I took of the possum as her computer backdrop for the next few months because she enjoyed trolling me at times.

What's the lesson here? Clinical life is full of strange, unexpected events and there's absolutely no way you can prepare for everything this job will throw at you. If someone had asked me during my training how I would problem-solve a wildlife invasion at work, I would probably have considered assessing them for psychosis. But when I share this story, my clinician friends inevitably tell me about other bizarre situations they've experienced: "That time a client took their shoe off and threw it at me" or "The time a patient brought bed bugs into the office and one jumped off his hat." Here's my best advice about this type of situation: when something odd happens, take a breath. Seek help, whether this is from your dad, another practitioner on site, or a good friend. Take a minute afterwards to settle yourself. And know that no matter how stressful you find that moment, it will probably make a really good story down the line.

On cursing

Cursing in therapy – should you ever do it? Should you only do it with certain clients or in certain settings? And, most importantly, which words are permitted and which ones are off-limits? The answer to all these excellent questions is "it depends." I'm Canadian by nationality and I'm given to understand that we as a people are more apt to use profanity than Americans, though I suspect we trail the Australians by a wide margin (Seidel, 2022). This section is especially culturally specific and your mileage may vary. I don't remember touching on this issue in my classes, but my professors didn't use these words during class or supervision so I graduated with a strong sense of "don't do it" even though no one had told me so explicitly. That's a fair default position and probably the safest stance to take in your early years as you develop your clinical acumen. You certainly wouldn't want to damage an alliance with a client by offending them early on in the relationship with your word choices.

However, consider also that clients use strong words to describe deeply painful situations. What signal do we give them if we deliberately temper their word choices or tone down the descriptions of their situations? If you don't achieve the correct balance, it can be terribly invalidating, and research has shown that swearing may help clients to see therapists as credible, authentic, trustworthy, non-judgmental, and caring (Williams & Uebel, 2021). I've had supervisors suggest that swearing is okay, but clinicians should wait until the client goes first. However, in practice, I've noticed that clients may not go first due to misplaced beliefs around the "allowability" of swearing in therapy and the implicit power hierarchy in the therapeutic relationship. I have, occasionally, "gone first" to break the ice; on these occasions, I have stayed closer to the mild-to-moderate end of the spectrum rather than the "extremely spicy" end. Always keep in mind differences related to gender, age, culture, race, and any other factors that could colour the situation and change perceptions of language use.

That being said, you will likely run into supervisors or managers who are not okay with cursing of any type. I once had a manager who told me she didn't appreciate my use of the word "shit." No problem...until a few weeks later, she called me into her office to explain that "damn" was also unacceptable. Please note that the hospital clinic where we worked was located in the downtown area of a major city and everyone in that setting – patients, family members, and healthcare professionals – was tough as nails. "Damn" was probably the most gentle profanity ever uttered by anyone in that setting. Anyway, due to cultural and linguistic differences, this manager was not familiar with the idiom "clusterf***" so I shortened it to "cluster" and used that to describe clinical situations when appropriate (i.e., "There's a real cluster happening in the ICU today"); this was considered acceptable and we both lived, if not happily, at least peacefully ever after. Get creative when necessary!

Using the doctor title, if you have it

Some of you may conclude your professional training with a "doctor" title. Should you insist that therapy clients use it and correct them if they don't? For me, I don't like the formality of the title and the sense of distance it creates between me and the client: it makes me uncomfortable that the power dynamic is implicitly reinforced every time the client addresses me. I also don't like the possibility of creating confusion about the scope of my practice, especially with clients whom I might meet only briefly ("No, I can't prescribe you benzos"). On the other hand, I want to support minoritized colleagues, who spend years fighting to be acknowledged and respected in their workplaces, and this could include the correct use of their titles. I've heard enough stories of racialized physicians presumed to be janitorial staff that I don't want to reinforce any part of that system through my choices. Telling your clients that they don't have to call you "doctor" may undermine the efforts of your colleagues to use the title that they've earned; while I don't believe in excessive formality, I do believe in solidarity.

Like the rest of this chapter, there's no good answer to this one (also, sorry, no refunds). Some of my clients used "Dana" and others stuck with "Dr. Ménard." The students to whom I provide clinical supervision usually refer to me as "doctor," though I expect they have different nicknames for private use amongst themselves. The one I definitely shut down from all parties is "Dr. Dana," which so many people felt compelled to use because of the hilarious alliteration but to me evokes images of well-known professional charlatans (e.g., "Dr. Phil", "Dr. Oz", or "Dr. Laura"). Keep in mind that some clients might prefer to use your title, to maintain a sense of formality and to reinforce their trust in you as the expert.

If you do decide to use the title, keep it to work settings and other situations when you want to flex your authority muscles (e.g., arguments with your cell phone company). I strongly recommend that you do *not* use it when booking airline tickets, or you may be called upon to perform CPR or deliver a baby mid-flight.

Accepting gifts

Clients bringing gifts to me has been a rare issue in my career, which suggests (1) it's not a common practice with the client populations and settings where I've worked and (2) I've been working in all the wrong places. Receiving gifts from clients is another professional situation where the "slippery" slope argument is routinely brought out, with some clinicians suggesting that accepting any kind of gift could lead to further boundary violations. I expect that most clinical relationships that did end in horrifying boundary violations probably started with something innocent like a coffee or a hug but I don't think the converse is true, that most coffees eventually lead to sex, in much the same way that most heroin users probably did start with marijuana but most marijuana users do not graduate to heroin.

In my experience, clients are most likely to bring gifts to a termination session, which makes the situation more complicated because you won't have much time to process the issue together if there's some kind of problem. Most ethical codes governing clinical practice have guidelines about accepting gifts from clients, with the general rule being that they must be of "token" value only (College of Psychologists of Ontario, 2017). In theory, this seems like a great idea; in practice, how are we to know what counts as token for the client or the therapist? Keep in mind also that gifts have very different meanings in different cultures – I have heard Middle Easterners reference gifts of jewelry as "just a little gold" but you might see it differently. Most of the gifts I have received from clients were flowers, drawings, and cards – clearly tokens but definitely of great value to me. Handmade gifts that require considerable energy on the part of the clients (e.g., knitting, paintings) might also fall into that category and many of us would not consider that gift to be a "token" given the time invested to their creation. A past supervisor of mine once accepted a bottle of wine that she presumed to be of token value; in fact, as she later discovered, the client's family was quite wealthy and the bottle was well over $200. Unfortunately, this meant that she could not add this wine to her regular dinnertime rotation. If you have concerns about the value or intent of the gift, you can always say no and cite your setting's cruel and draconian policies, but I would recommend that you then spend a few minutes ensuring your client doesn't feel shamed or rejected. Look also for creative solutions. A colleague of mine who regularly received gift cards from grateful clients had a policy of using them to buy items for her practice (e.g., therapeutic toys) that could benefit future clients.

Now and then, I've had a client bring me a hot beverage to a session but it's uncommon. On these occasions, you will have the opportunity to process whether it was a just thoughtful gesture or whether it might reveal some need for them to take care of you; you can then explore how that might apply to other relationships in their lives. Just last week, I had a student come to my office hours with a to-go cup in both hands, explaining that the coffee shop had accidentally made her first drink wrong; however, in this case, she elected to keep both for herself.

Conclusion

There are no clear answers to most questions about professionalism, and every supervisor or manager is going to have a different opinion. The issue as I see it is that many people in the field mistake their personal set of choices for the objective "right way" in which all these issues must be resolved. Whether you agree or not, follow the rules for where you work and think critically about the ones that you think are relevant to your future practice and the ones that you think aren't a great fit for you. Most importantly, pay attention to the impact of your choices on your relationships with clients and how you feel. And watch out for attempted wildlife invasions of your office, you never know when those might happen.

Part 2

The "grown-up" years

Chapter 7

Outpatient settings

Throughout my graduate training and afterwards, I worked in a variety of different outpatient settings, including private practice, hospital clinics, and post-secondary student counselling centres. Depending on where you train, you may work in all of these places at some point or focus on one in particular. Each has their own unique characteristics and skills required for working with that patient population and each has their own unique set of lessons to take away.

Private practice

Depending on your training program, you may get lots of experience working in private practices before you graduate, a little taste of it, or possibly nothing at all; I fell into the last group but my first real "adult" job post-graduation was in a private practice. My very first client in that new setting walked in with concerns around anxiety: they worried all day every day, experienced painful muscle tension, suffered from headaches and insomnia, and felt constantly on edge. A quick assessment revealed that their daily routine included at least one full pot of coffee, two packs of cigarettes, and several alcoholic beverages. For those of you who don't care to revisit organic chemistry, caffeine plus nicotine plus mild alcohol withdrawal symptoms equals lots of anxiety. I suggested that part of their treatment would likely involve finding alternate strategies to address the needs that were currently being filled by all these substances; the client instead requested that I give them a prescription for anti-anxiety medication (i.e., another chemical to add to the churning mix of anxiety soup inside of them). I explained that as a psychologist, I could only provide talk therapy, but I was willing to help them connect with a psychiatrist or medical practitioner to address their pharmacological needs. I got a skeptical look in reply and the client never came back, which certainly felt like an illustrious start to a new chapter in my professional life. Thankfully, private practice life improved from there.

DOI: 10.4324/9781003355366-10

Finding the balance. One of the main issues I experienced in transitioning from no-fee outpatient work to private practice was finding the right balance between assessing and treating clients. I had received most of my clinical training in settings where you could take three or more sessions to assess and complete testing, and then offer an additional session of feedback before starting treatment. When services are free, I find that clients have more patience for this kind of delay in starting the intervention piece of the work; when services are paid, clients need to make the most of their limited resources and start feeling better a lot earlier if they're going to come back. You don't have the luxury of spending that much time on information-gathering and case conceptualization – you have to start helping right from the get-go.

I will freely admit that my early work in private practice involved both types of mistakes you can make in this situation: in some cases, I delayed the start of the intervention phase too long and in others, I started it too early. Neither feels particularly good and both can result in clients terminating therapy prematurely. I had a client come in once with serious substance use disorder symptoms who was worried about the impact this was having on their child. This issue was a generational one: the client's parent had suffered from the same substance use disorder symptoms and it had severely affected my client as a child. Naturally, I wanted to explore the experience of intergenerational trauma and the impact on the client of visiting the same stress on their child as had been visited on them. Instead, the client wanted me to give them "coping skills" and didn't want to address the past or their repetition of trauma in their own family. I explained that generic coping skills without a personalized understanding of the client and their circumstances would be no better than sharing a 10-item "list"-icle from a website, which they could likely find for themselves; however, the client insisted so we spent part of our third session identifying possible "coping skills." Unsurprisingly, that was our last meeting.

I wish I could give you some exact numbers here about how to organize your time in private practice but it will depend on the client, their problems, and their financial situation. It will be important to identify and discuss time-related challenges as soon as possible and adjust your plans as needed. For example, if a couple came in and told me they only had coverage for six sessions, instead of having one session assessing the couple, one session with each individual, and then a session to review the assessment and discuss goals, I'd try to condense that whole process down to two sessions. Do your best to explain that therapy requires getting to know one another but also throw out some actionable strategies from day 1 to make the most of the time they have. Keep in mind that you can still provide a lot of help in a limited number of meetings. Can you completely change a client's life? Maybe not. Can you help them carve out some tiny area of flexibility to make a change that could grow over time? Absolutely.

Handling payments. If your training experiences were concentrated in settings that offered free psychotherapy, taking money or credit cards and then handing over receipts may feel pretty strange: "I hope I just helped you out but either way, it'll be $180." Luckily, in my first private practice job, we had an old-fashioned credit card imprinter, also known as a "ZipZap machine," a "click-clack machine," or a "Knuckle Buster." In addition to taking credit card imprints, this device also served an important role as a payment-processing ice breaker. Younger clients required an explanation as to what it was and what it did; older clients marvelled at the device, telling me that they had not seen such a machine in decades. On the odd occasion, I would injure myself with the machine ("Knuckler Buster" indeed) and clients would either empathize or laugh, which also provided helpful clinical information. A year or so into the job, my boss did finally upgrade to a smartphone-based app, possibly as a result of my repeated allusions to danger pay.

I wouldn't go so far as to recommend acquiring one for your own practice but it does help to have something you can joke about, a few stock lines or some kind of ritual to help you get past the initial awkwardness of taking payment from clients, if that is part of your role. For example, "We've come to the end of our hour. Do you want to book another appointment? And how should I spell your name for the receipt?"

Private practice loneliness. Depending on the specifics of your private practice set-up, working in these settings can be a very lonely experience (Adames et al., 2022; Melamed et al., 2001). In one practice, I shared my office with another associate and so I literally never met her – I was in on Mondays and Tuesdays, she was in on Wednesdays and Thursdays. Our entire relationship revolved around repositioning the office garbage can. At another practice, the clinicians all worked different schedules and took different lunch breaks, so interactions were limited to quick catch-ups when clients were late. During those years, there were days where the only people I interacted with were clients, which began to take a toll over time: unlike coworkers, clients aren't going to ask about your child's dance recital or the half-marathon you ran last weekend. Even if everyone is just being polite, those brief connections still add up over the day and you miss them when they're not available.

Here are a few thoughts on addressing and combating private practice loneliness:

• Make sure you get plenty of social interactions in other ways: a yoga class, running group, amateur drama troupe, garage band punk rock group – whatever floats your boat. Just make sure you have the opportunity to talk to people who aren't your clients routinely.

- Cultivate acquaintanceships to break up your practice day. In one job, I fell into the habit of going to the shopping mall next door to grab a hot tea midday and became friendly with the barista who worked there. Was it a deep and intimate relationship filled with lots of sharing? No. Did she ask about my recent half-marathon? Yes. This might have had something to do with the tips I left, but I cherished the relationship nonetheless.
- Join a professional association of psychologists. Whether it's local, state/provincial or federal, find a relevant professional interest group and get involved. Go to the meetings and talks and take advantage of the free snacks that these events typically feature. If there isn't one for your city, consider starting one.

Private practice stereotypes. Some members of the mental health community endorse some very inaccurate and biased beliefs about private practice work. The expression I've heard most often in connection with this client population is "the worried well" meaning that these people are not *really* in need of services but are presenting to therapy with "normal" life problems (e.g., Catterson et al., 1997; Gray et al., 2020; Dembowsky, 2016). I find statements of this type very troubling.

First of all, there's actually quite a range of mental health issues and severity represented in the problems of private practice clients; in these settings, I saw severe mood and anxiety disorders, debilitating chronic pain, crushing grief, and every flavour of family dysfunction you could imagine. I saw clients with long trauma histories, clients who had misused every substance under the sun, and some presenting problems that I've never seen before or since. I suspect this has a lot to do with the relative absence of services available through the publicly-funded systems – where else are people going to go for help? If you wind up working in a setting of this type, don't imagine that your days of challenging cases are behind you, and do try to maintain your academic library membership because you're likely to need it.

Moreover, the belief that some clients are only "worried" also implies that people who have mild symptoms or medium symptoms don't deserve treatment when there are people out there who have severe symptoms. You may recall your mother using a similar argument when she told you to finish your dinner plate because there were starving children in other parts of the world; this is flawed logic as applied to any social issue, but I find it particularly egregious when it comes from mental health professionals. We all know that it may not take much for someone with medium symptoms to experience very significant symptoms indeed: the loss of a job, an illness, the end of a relationship, the death of a friend or family member. And finally, don't people with medium symptoms deserve to feel better too?

In summary, (1) private practice work may include lots of different presenting issues of varying degrees of severity and (2) some clinicians need to work on their manners.

Hospital outpatients

I find that clinicians usually fall into one of two camps: people who love a specific client group or problem and want to focus primarily on that kind of work (e.g., trans clients, patients with eating disorders) and people who need more diversity in their practice. I'm definitely the second kind, but I know a lot of very happy clinicians in that first group; if this is you, specialized outpatient clinics might be the ideal work setting. Over the years, I trained and worked in several different hospital outpatient clinics including both the psychiatric type and the "regular" type (where psychological issues were often secondary to medical issues). In all of these settings, the services were free but eligibility for psychotherapy depended on presenting with a specific mental and/or physical health issue or falling into a specific age bracket (e.g., late adolescence/early adulthood). Each of these settings offered their own particular challenges and their own special learning experiences.

Outpatient challenges. Having said that outpatient clinics are for people who like to specialize, keep in mind that clients rarely present with just the main issue served by the clinic; just because your clinic or department specializes in anxiety, for example, doesn't mean that you won't be assessing and addressing a whole host of other issues. In one setting, I saw so many mood-disordered clients who also had concurrent symptoms of psychosis (e.g., auditory hallucinations) that my supervisor joked that I should have gotten credit for a completely different placement. Clients in these settings will often qualify for multiple diagnoses in the same chapter of the Diagnostic and Statistical Manual (DSM) as well as other chapters, on top of possible physical health concerns and the usual family/relationship/job/friend/financial troubles. So don't worry that your other clinical muscles are going to atrophy, you'll still be doing plenty of work on other issues.

Another challenge related to clients who present in these settings is that many have been in treatment for some time, and they may be understandably skeptical that you have anything new, interesting or helpful to offer that they haven't heard from a long line-up of similarly well-meaning mental health professionals. That's okay; in fact, it would be genuinely surprising, not to mention clinically noteworthy, if they weren't at least a little bit skeptical. Here's a useful mantra: "I could be the right therapist at the right time." Sometimes the stars finally line up for the client and you're the lucky clinician who gets to benefit from this. Similarly, these clients may be quite familiar with some basic therapeutic concepts (e.g., thought records, relaxation strategies) and assure you vehemently that these strategies have not improved their problems in the slightest. Don't be put off by this. Even if you say nothing to them that some other therapist hasn't said before, or even 10 times before, the client themselves is always in a different place in their life: they may finally be ready to hear and implement something for the first time. You might be the first person to use the specific words they really needed to properly grasp the technique. Don't be tempted to skip the fundamentals even if a client claims familiarity, but definitely do spend some time trying to understand why these approaches may not have worked in the past and more broadly, what was or was not helpful about past therapeutic experiences.

Symptom severity implications. Often, a prerequisite for clients to be seen in such outpatient clinics is a certain level of symptom severity or impairment; as a result, clients in these settings are very likely to be taking one or more medications. In some cases, clients were taking so many prescriptions that I was surprised they didn't rattle as they walked. I've often found in these cases that different medications are prescribed by each member on their treatment team, who may not have checked what the client is already taking or touched base with other providers to coordinate care (Bokhof & Junius-Walker, 2016; Smith et al., 2010). It is important that someone on the team makes sure that all these medications are not interacting with one another chemically and producing additional symptoms rather than controlling them, as clients may end up on drug combinations that seem to "contradict" one another (e.g., laxatives and anti-diarrhea meds) or medications that are not advisable to combine. For example, some pain management medications also include caffeine to counteract daytime sleepiness; clients on these medications might consider moving to different pain management medications rather than simply adding sleeping pills on top of their current prescriptions. Clients who experience symptoms of mania while taking Selective Serotonin Reuptake Inhibitors (SSRIs) may actually have bipolar disorder, not major depressive disorder, and need to be on a mood stabilizer instead. May I suggest that you make a friend like a pharmacist, a psychiatrist, or a physician to talk you through the impact of various drug combinations? Yes, as a mental health person, that's not your job (and may bring on horrible flashbacks to chemistry class) but you can at least gently encourage your client to bring the list to someone who does specialize in such issues to double-check.

Depending on the severity of their illness, outpatients in these types of settings may have already experienced disclosures of confidential information in order to activate safety plans such as being involuntarily hospitalized to address suicidality. Such plans are critically important and they may be the reason that the client is still alive to be sitting in your office;

however, these events, depending on how they are handled, can breed significant mistrust with healthcare providers and prevent them from consciously providing information about their suicide risk (Blanchard & Farber, 2020; Duncan et al., 2015). Unsurprisingly, many clients don't enjoy suddenly losing their fundamental freedoms (often including losing access to all electronic devices) to spend an unknown amount of time sleeping on uncomfortable mattresses and eating hospital food. Some may have experienced the use of chemical and/or physical restraints against their will, and there may be challenges or difficulties due to the collateral damage of these events in the rest of their lives (e.g., job loss, damage to relationships). If a previous provider has had to breach confidentiality to protect a patient from harm, address it early: ask how the disclosure was handled, their experiences as an inpatient, the impact to the rest of their life, and, most importantly, how the two of you could handle such an event based on what the client learned from that event.

Student counselling centres

From internship onwards, I spent several years working in university counselling centres. During that time, I went from "basically a student myself" years old to "clients feel compelled to explain pop culture to me" years old. I suspect this phenomenon only gets worse if you spend a significant amount of your career in such a setting: as a clinician, you will get older and older but your clients will remain in their late teens and early 20s and let me assure you, there are no clients who will make you feel your age quite so keenly as university students, who are complete monsters in that regard. They will refer to "old movies" that came out when you were a teen (in my case, *Titanic*). They will miss all your references to classic sitcoms but mock you ruthlessly if you are unfamiliar with the latest Tik Tok influencers and YouTube stars. However, apart from the relentless reminders of the aging process, I find them a very appealing population to work with and enjoyed those jobs immensely.

Student counseling stereotypes. I completed my pre-doctoral internship at a student counseling centre located at a fancy-pants university; before I started, I was told by several people that most of the students who attended that school were spoiled, rich, white kids who would come to me to complain about exam stress and other mild problems. Nothing could have been further from the truth, both at that setting and other counselling centres where I eventually found myself.

For starters, the clients at student counselling centres came from a variety of different demographic groups, including a substantial proportion from marginalized and minoritized identities: I saw students from all different racial, ethnic, and socioeconomic backgrounds, as well as first-generation students who had no family or friends to help them navigate the process of higher education. I worked with students who had immigrated to Canada, students whose families had immigrated to Canada, and international students from virtually every continent. And then there was the variety of presenting problems: I saw clients with severe eating disorders, psychotic symptoms, major mood and anxiety disorders, serious trauma, significant health concerns, and every kind of relationship and family dysfunction. I worked with a refugee from a war-torn area, who described holding a neighbour in their arms while the person died of multiple bullet wounds. I saw a student who had found their roommate after a suicide attempt the previous evening, halfway through the final exam period. I worked with more than one client who had recently found out that their fathers had a second, secret family. I saw clients who were stuck in elaborate lies to their families about their academic progress or who they were dating and were terrified that they would be disowned or worse should these secrets be discovered. The one exception to all these deeply serious issues (and I do mean the only one) was the student who scheduled a session to complain that their friend had borrowed their $300 trucker's hat without asking. Please note that at the time, I was making the equivalent of $14/hour after completing 11 years of university. All this to say, if you are working or plan to work in such a setting, feel confident that you will get both depth and breadth in your exposure to different kinds of clients and different kinds of issues: post-secondary populations are diverse in all senses of the word.

Multidisciplinary work on campus. As a psychotherapist, you can't escape multidisciplinary work – it's everywhere! Except instead of physicians, nurses, and occupational therapists, in student counselling centres, you will need to liaise with academic staff and professors. Students in distress often approach staff or faculty first; unfortunately, few staff members or professors receive appropriate training to prepare them for the stories students may share or the state of emotional dysregulation in which they may present (Ménard et al., 2021). You may find yourself with a freaked-out professor knocking on your office door to talk about an email they just received from a student disclosing suicidal ideation, or a staff member calling to find out where on campus they can send someone in the middle of an active panic attack. You may also need to connect with different divisions on campus to help students get support for the various other life concerns affecting their mental health, which may include medical staff, the student accommodations office, the housing office, or the student academic success centre. Some universities even have established multidisciplinary teams including mental health experts, campus police, case managers, and residence staff to assist students in crisis who are exhibiting behaviours troubling to other campus community members.

Knowing what's out there and sharing that information may be a surprisingly large component of your work. Resources on campus are often siloed and people working in specific departments or faculties may not be aware of what services are offered centrally, and vice versa; professors and even upper-level administrators like deans may not be aware of what's available to students (Ménard et al., in press). Part of your job will be connecting students to these resources, but another part of your job is likely to be educating staff and faculty about resources so that they can make the connections too. You can compare yourself to an old-fashioned telephone switchboard operator, but I've found that students often don't understand that reference (and then mock me).

Managing your own reactions. Working in student counselling settings as a former or current student yourself may bring up some strong emotional reactions in you, possibly including some over-identification with your clients and their problems. Whether you have recently graduated from your own program or are still in the thick of it, I strongly advise you to identify and at least try to start processing your own school-related neuroses. I know you've got it – no one graduates from a psychotherapy training program without at least some emotional baggage. The clients you see in student counselling centres are very likely to share stories and experiences that remind you of the worst moments of your own education, from toxic professors to public speaking disasters to traumatic breakups during midterm week (this is nicknamed the "Turkey dump" at some student counselling centres because it usually happens when everyone goes home to celebrate Thanksgiving). This can be very challenging to address without descending into a complete countertransference mess if you are fresh out of that same hell yourself. Consider the lowlights of your educational career and be prepared to help others navigate those same snake pits, otherwise you may find yourself over-identifying with the students who are struggling to manage, oh I don't know, receiving an A- in their graduate-level trauma class despite their colleague who did the other half of the presentation receiving an A. I'm not bitter.

Your emotional reaction to working with students might also include some level of wishful thinking – the mind loves telling you that the grass is greener on the other side. If you're like me, you might wonder what your life would have been like if you had chosen some other field of study and pursued a different profession. Working with different kinds of students will allow you to see the road not taken in a very clear way, which can be very helpful as you will see both the upside and the very real downsides of the choices you didn't make. Were you a quiet, studious, indoorsy student? Of course you were. Don't worry, your party animal clients are here to show you what life would look like if you had gone out to clubs and bars three nights a week. Here's a hint: it often involves sitting for exams very, very hungover. Did you contemplate becoming a varsity athlete? These clients will show you the challenges associated with travelling every weekend, training two hours a day, and still getting your assignments done. Did you perhaps think that business or medicine or environmental science would be a more exciting major? These clients will show you the challenges of these areas, ranging from incessant groupwork (business), to mandatory chemistry classes (medicine), to getting bitten by the animals you study (environmental science). No other group of clients has ever made me feel so good about my own choices in life, with the possible exception of couple therapy (see Chapter 8).

General outpatient concerns

Running into clients: it's going to happen. Running into clients in public is always awkward and fraught, depending on where you are, who you are with, and what you are doing. For the first few years of my clinical practice, I had an unusual run of good luck about not seeing clients in public. I did one time wave enthusiastically when I saw a client at a bus stop before I realized I shouldn't be doing that, but the client waved back and I don't think anyone else at the bus stop thought anything of the interaction other than "Look at those two dorks."

My run of good luck ended while I was running errands one day with my husband; more specifically, we were at a Bulk Barn. If you're not familiar with the joy that is Bulk Barn[1], it's a chain of Canadian bulk food stores characterized by large clear plastic bins filled with everything from pasta to almonds to spices. More importantly, it sells a wide array of candy. We were standing at the cash register clutching our oversized bags of gummy worms when a current client standing behind us in line started talking to me in a very familiar way: "Hey Dana. How are you doing?" I tried to answer as non-chalantly as I could without revealing personal details on either side and without drawing my husband's attention, which was both difficult and awkward. The cashier slowed to a snail's pace. My husband looked quizzically between me and the client, the client looked quizzically at my husband, and I could tell both were wondering why I wasn't making an introduction. Eventually, the cashier completed the world's slowest checkout and we all went on our merry way, though my happiness about

1 For readers outside of Canada, you need to understand that Bulk Barn is an *institution* to its devoted fans. In the early days of the COVID-19 pandemic, the Arkells, a popular Canadian rock band, posted a worried tweet asking whether Bulk Barn was considered an essential service and would therefore be allowed to remain open. The answer was yes on both counts.

the bag of gummy worms was greatly diminished. The client and I discussed the awkwardness of this encounter in the next session and they took no offense to my admittedly strange and impolite behaviour. Some time later, as a completely random topic of discussion, I explained to my husband that hypothetically, were we ever to run into a client in public, I would not be introducing him so he should just politely wander off during such an interaction. To be fair, of all the places where you could run into a client, Bulk Barn is not the most embarrassing (that would be a toss up between the locker room at the gym and a sex store), and I would have cheerfully self-disclosed my ardent admiration for the store had a client asked in session. I've since run into clients on other occasions, but I've often found that they have failed to recognize me; if clients are used to seeing you in therapy clothes in a therapy office, the brain often struggles to identify that same person in a different setting.

Running into clients in public is not an "if it happens" but a "when it happens" kind of scenario. You're certainly welcome to discuss what you might do if you see one another in public during the intake; this might even be advisable if you work in a small town, belong to the same small subculture or some other circumstance makes it extra-likely that you will run into one another outside of the clinical setting. Another good option is to include a short write-up about public encounters in your intake paperwork, if you are able to do so. Most clinicians I know use some variation on "I won't acknowledge you, but you are free to acknowledge me." You might also consider, as I did when working in student counselling centres, avoiding bars where undergraduates are known to congregate, not only because you might run into clients but mostly because at your age, you probably don't want to be going out for the night to the same places that the undergrads go.

Managing patient nudity. There are many sections of this book where I could have included the following section on client nudity, but I chose to include it here, partly because so much of it happened in various outpatient settings but mostly because this was one of the more shocking aspects of work in these locations. In an inpatient setting, it's not altogether surprising that a patient who has seriously impairing symptoms and is on heavy medication might lose track of who you are amongst a sea of other white coats on their treatment team and try to show you their rash. It was quite a bit more surprising to me when clients in private practice tried to show me their rashes, and they did – routinely. At least I'm not alone – please see Kahr (2005) for a hilarious description of his reaction to a patient who walked into his office and immediately pulled off her caftan:

Of course, having worked in long-stay psychogeriatric institutions and on acute psychiatric wards, I had seen many distressed patients running around at one time or another without clothing, but always on the open wards, with fleets of house officers and nurses in hot pursuit.

How many medical professionals are required to make up a "fleet," I wonder?

My first brush with client nudity came early in my training. I had completed an intake session with a new client and my supervisor's first question to me was, "Did they show you their axe scar?" "No!" I said, aghast, "Is that something this person is likely to do?" "Yes," said my supervisor, "because they've done it with everyone else they've seen so far. You'll know they're about to do it when they reach down to pull up their pant leg." Sure enough, the client made a move towards their feet at our next session but luckily, I was able to gently redirect them (shockingly, the event that led to the axe scar was not at all the focus of our treatment). In the years since that moment, I saw a surprising amount of skin for a clinical psychologist; I say "surprising" because in this profession, I was genuinely expecting to see very little skin at all. In some cases, clients appeared to be confused about my educational background and a brief reiteration of who I was did the trick ("Not that kind of doctor!"). In other cases, clients with injuries or chronic pain were literally showing me where it hurt; gentle recommendations to bring this up with more-qualified members of their treatment team helped but sometimes I was called on to admire the kinesio tape applied by their physiotherapists. Some clients wanted to show me where their next tattoo would be located; I'm still unclear why they couldn't just point above their clothes, and I suspect boundary issues may have been at play. Other incidents included new mothers who brought their babies to session and breastfed them rather than cancel the appointment – a reasonable choice for a group of people usually in dire need of support – and university students wearing especially avant-garde fashions, a much less reasonable choice for people who were going to class immediately afterwards.

Client nudity presents two main challenges: (1) how to gently, empathically, warmly, compassionately tell patients to cover up in order to maintain professional boundaries and (2) how to appropriately document this unrequested nudity in session notes. I don't know whether these kinds of situations happened to any of my professors but none of them ever covered sample wording that one could use in such a situation. Maybe I'm just lucky? Anyway, the main focus of your response should be to kindly reiterate the professional nature of your relationship, emphasize the focus on dignity within psychotherapy, and gently advise them to cover up. The important thing is to tell, not ask: "I'm going to need you to put your shirt back down please" rather than "Could you put your shirt back down, please?" If you make it an option, plenty of clients will tell you that they are not bothered and are happy to continue the session with their bare chest on display. A constipated hospital patient once offered to have our session while they sat on the commode and strained – I declined. If necessary, you can always blame the draconian licensing bodies and their unaccountable fixation on professionalism in psychotherapy relationships (those weirdos).

The other challenge to this situation is how to describe this situation in a session note and yes, you definitely need to do this second part to cover your butt – in this case, figuratively. You want to make it clear that you were not the one who was inviting any level of nudity. "Patient showed me where he will be having his next tattoo placed by lifting his shirt. This was not requested of him," should do the trick.

Wrapping up therapy. In 2016, I was working at two private practices when my husband landed his dream job in a city two hours away; there-fore, in the spring of that year, I ended therapy with about 50 different clients within the space of a month. I'd wrapped up placements and left jobs previously, but this was a particularly striking experience because it involved so many clients over such a short span of time. I think I saw every possible emotional reaction to the end of the therapy relationship. Some had the more "expected" reaction: we both expressed sadness about part-ing and wished one another well. A few gave me cards or other tokens of affection. Other clients seemed to shrug it off, like I had told them it would rain later in the week: not what they had in mind, but not a big issue (ouch – there goes my saviour complex). A few clients no-showed to their last session, which is not an uncommon reaction in people who struggle with strong emotion. One client ended up sobbing uncontrollably and was probably the last person I would have expected to respond in this way.

Be prepared for anything at termination. You'll find out how your cli-ents deal with loss, sadness, anxiety, and interpersonal challenges. Ending therapy is a fantastic way to get a lot more data about your clients; unfor-tunately, you probably won't be able to use it with them. If you are the one doing the terminating because you are leaving, make sure you tell your clients with a few sessions to spare to process this transition as well. And, make sure you give yourself some time to process your own feelings of sadness and loss as needed too.

Conclusion

Outpatient work comes in all different forms and flavours. Depending on your setting, you may be surprised by the diversity you see in the clients and in their presenting problems; do feel free to ignore uninformed com-ments from others about what kind of clients they expect you'll be seeing.

Unfortunately, opportunities to work in publicly funded clinics offering treatment to outpatients are few and far-between in Canada these days, and unlikely to be full-time when they are available. I am hopeful that ongoing mental health advocacy will see increased funding for such clinics so that jobs in these settings will be more available within the profession.

Chapter 8

Couple therapy

Not everyone who pursues psychotherapy as a career will work with couples, but clients' romantic relationships will likely be relevant across all forms of therapy. Even if you never do therapy with more than one person in the room, it's good to have an understanding of the dynamics that keep people stuck in dysfunctional patterns of interaction with the person they love most in the world. That being said, couple therapy[1] is some of the most challenging and difficult work I ever did, and I'm including in this comparison my time working in a prison (people mandated into treatment) and seeing patients at a major trauma hospital (people with recent gunshot wounds).

Please note that the term "couples" in this chapter is intended to refer to all types of couples regardless of sexual orientation, marital status, or monogamy, though I will note also that most of the couples I worked with were heterosexual and, at least on paper, monogamous. Although the content of the conflict may differ across different types of couples, the conflict process of dysfunctional couples has more in common than otherwise (Kurdek, 2006; Peplau & Fingerhut, 2007).

Buckle up

Couple therapy is an entirely different rodeo altogether from individual therapy, and yes, I chose the word "rodeo" deliberately: I often found myself feeling like a clown trying to prevent arguments in the therapy room from getting completely out of hand and occasionally, I failed spectacularly. When I started doing couple therapy, my supervisor at the time told me, "You know how you've learned to sit back, listen carefully, and

1 And if you're wondering whether it should be "couple's therapy" or "couples therapy" or "couple therapy", there is a right answer – it's couple therapy (see Caldwell, 2018 for a more detailed grammatical explanation).

DOI: 10.4324/9781003355366-11

reflect back to slow your clients down? Yeah, you absolutely can't do that in couple therapy. You've got to step in before things escalate or get out of control."

Here's the main difference, as I see it: in individual therapy, someone is sitting across from you telling a story about the pain they've experienced. Whether it's about an event in the past or a relationship that exists outside the therapy room, it's a story, and therefore at least somewhat at arm's length. In couple therapy, the pain is not a story and it is not at arm's length – it is happening live and in-person, and it is coming from the person sitting next to them on the couch. Instead of someone describing "That comment my partner made last week that hurt my feelings quite badly," you might see that comment happen right in front of you. This has a few implications:

(1) Your assessments are likely to be much, much more accurate because you can actually collect data yourself. Instead of someone describing their typical response in a conflict, you'll get to hear it directly and observe the ensuing interaction.
(2) The emotion is live in session so your opportunity to teach people to talk, behave, or think differently, even when they're having intense feelings, is greatly enhanced. This is *in vivo* learning at its finest.
(3) Pursuant to #2, you can lose control of a session so much faster and with far less warning. I was often genuinely surprised at how quickly a couple can go from reasonably respectful conversation to cursing one another's ancestors, but when you've been having some version of the same argument for years, a seemingly innocuous phrase may actually be quite loaded. Stay alert!

Some of the most colourful and intense sessions over my entire career have involved couples. For example, the pair who took a pregnancy test in the bathroom outside my office right before our regular session (it was positive), the pair who got into an actual physical scuffle in my office, or the pair who described a history of infidelity, with each other and every other previous partner, so convoluted and graphic they made Tiger Woods look like a monk (this was the same pair who asked for a 50% discount on our usual hourly rate).

All this to say that many clinicians who work with couples will schedule one or two at a maximum per day and fill the rest of their time with individual sessions in order to preserve their stamina for what can be genuinely taxing clinical work. I once came back from vacation to find that my boss, someone with whom I generally had an excellent relationship, had put me down for five couple sessions in one day. A quick discussion established that this was a scheduling accident and not a passive-aggressive attempt to get me to quit but I did wonder for a few minutes.

Real clients are nothing like textbook clients – couple edition

We've all heard that old chestnut: "There are lies, damned lies, and statistics." I posit to you that there exists a fourth set of lies – fake client dialogues in textbooks. This is definitely true for individual clients (see Chapter 2 p. 30); however, I think it's far more egregious when it comes to couples. Let me illustrate with an example:

Typical textbook couple conversation

Elaine:	I find it really frustrating when you take your clothes off at night and leave them on the floor. I want our house to be tidy. (softly)
Therapist:	Jim, it sounds like Elaine is trying to communicate that the socks on the floor evoke a deeper emotional response for her. What do you feel when you hear her say that? (calmly)
Jim:	I feel bad. I understand that Elaine grew up in a chaotic, disorganized house and she found it very stressful. Even though our household is very different, I can see that the socks on the floor evoke bad memories for her. I will try to implement some process to ensure that I don't leave my clothes on the floor at night. (looks deeply into her eyes with a warm, empathic gaze)
Therapist:	Elaine, it sounds like Jim didn't realize that the problem with socks on the floor isn't *really* about socks on the floor. How do you feel when he says that? (gently)
Elaine:	It's so lovely to hear that. (voice breaks) I appreciate that, and I appreciate you, Jim. (Elaine tears up. Jim tears up. The therapist tears up. End scene with group hug).

Here's how I see that dialogue unfolding in real life:

Elaine:	Every goddamn night, you leave your socks on the goddam floor. What the hell is wrong with you, I've asked you a hundred times to just pick them up?! (high volume)
Therapist:	Jim, it sounds like Elaine is trying to communicate that the socks on the floor evoke a deeper emotional response for her. What do you feel when you hear her say that? (calmly)

Jim:	She needs to shut up about my socks. It's just socks, why does she have to be such a bitch about it?!! (animatedly)
Therapist:	Jim could we just pause for a second –
Elaine:	(interrupts) And another thing – he leaves his wet towel on the floor every morning after he showers and it drives me insane!! (Turns to him) Were you raised by wolves?!
Therapist:	Uh, hang on a sec – (desperately trying to regain control of the session)
Jim:	My towel?! Well what about your mother dropping by without calling every other day?! Like mother, like daughter! You're a pair of crazy bitches!! (shouting)
[couple shouts over one another, end scene]

I once attended a two-day training seminar about couple therapy; it was at a conference centre outside the airport, which should have been my first clue that this workshop would more closely approximate a multi-level-marketing initiation than a helpful educational experience. The facilitators were trying to illustrate an exercise on assessing couples' deeper values and how early life experiences can sometimes drive present-day conflicts. We watched a training video where the therapist asked both people in the couple to name their favourite type of tree. The male half of the couple replied with a long, drawn-out description of the plum tree that grew in his impoverished urban neighbourhood; during the summer, the fruit of that tree attracted all the children in the area to feast together and created a kind of harmony that was so lacking in their difficult circumstances. Meanwhile, the female half of the couple nodded slowly, tears in her eyes; clearly, she was re-evaluating her previous frustration about his tendency to fill up the dishwasher but not run it.

I'm not saying that this type of experience in couple therapy is impossible. I don't doubt couples like that are out there, somewhere, but if I judged the utility of my own sessions based on that example, I'd be ready to throw out my license and open up a bakery. Sometimes couples can calm down enough to have a conversation like that in session; more often, they're in so much pain and so emotionally dysregulated that a poorly timed question like, "What is your favourite tree and why?" could really wreck the alliance. Don't be hard on yourself if you don't see an opportunity for that sort of intervention and don't be too hard on your clients if they're not in the mood to consider what flavour of ice cream they would be if they had to choose.

Interrupt early, interrupt often

If you want to work with couples, you will need to work on your gentle, warm, empathic interrupting skills because you're going to be using them – a lot. Couple therapy often requires far more directiveness from the therapist than individual work (Fraenkel, 2019; Vansteenwegen, 1998), which can be a big change for clinicians who are used to sitting back, allowing the person to tell their story, and slowly processing and exploring the material. With couples, the emotion can get out of control quickly so you need to (1) nip these things in the bud and (2) clearly establish the precedent that you will be nipping things in the bud.

In the early sessions, you might want to let a conflict play out for a minute or two to see how the couple actually interacts and responds to one another but letting it go on much longer than that is inadvisable for a few reasons. Most couples have already caused each other significant pain and damage long before they make their way into your office with recurring arguments, and there's little value in allowing them to go through the motions of a conflict that has likely played out dozens if not hundreds of times already. They know this dance well (Johnson, 2019). There's also the issue of time: if you thought 50 minutes wasn't much time for an individual session, you're about to see just how short 50 minutes can really be. It can take a couple much longer to calm down and re-regulate, so allowing a conflict to build from a 2/10 to a 7/10 will take more time to recover from than a 7 out of 10 for an individual.

Here's a weird trick that I picked up from a supervisor, which is to say that he didn't teach me this directly, but I realized one day that he was doing it on me. This might have been unethical but it was certainly effective. At the end of supervision, he would gently smack his hands palm down on his thighs as a prelude to rising from his chair and moving back to the rest of his schedule; like Pavlov's dogs, I learned that the hand smacking motion presaged the end of our meeting. You can use this to your advantage in interrupting clients, both individuals and couples. Make a certain hand gesture every time you interrupt a couple: lean forward and put one hand on your knee right before you say, "I'm going to stop you there," or just hold your hand out palm forward (not unlike The Supremes singing "Stop in the name of love"). Over time and multiple repetitions, you should get to a point where you can just make the gesture and the couple will cease and desist. And don't be surprised by how often you use it, at least at first.

Checking your own values at the door

You may have strong beliefs about various relationship issues. You might believe some version of "once a cheater, always a cheater," and that relationships marred by infidelity are not salvageable. You may have strong feelings about the wisdom of sacrificing your own career in order to support a partner's career. You may think there is an ideal level of involvement by extended family, or that certain child-rearing practices are objectively better than others. This is definitely an example of my own values creeping in, but I was very surprised when I started this work at the topics that couples *didn't* discuss until they had already made major commitments to one another, including how to parent children from previous relationships, or the amount of financial debt each person was carrying. Remember, your clients may be learning something new and important about their partner at the exact same time you do, after they have made significant investments in the relationship like having children, buying real estate, or getting matching tattoos.

If you're planning to work with couples, try to identify these beliefs in yourself so that you can be ready to take a neutral stance if the issue comes up, or as neutral as possible. You may firmly believe that it is a bad idea to stay with a partner who has been unfaithful or that mothers-in-law should *not* be given a key to the marital home, but the couple sitting across from you may see the situation quite differently. Save your personal thoughts for debriefing with fellow couple therapists.

The individual sessions

It's recommended in most approaches to couple therapy to have individual sessions with each member of the couple (e.g., Jacobson et al., 2000; Johnson, 2019). In an ideal world, you'd want to have one joint session, two individual sessions, and then a summary session to synthesize information and set goals. When people only have a limited amount of insurance coverage for therapy – six sessions is not uncommon – I've sometimes split a single session in half in order to facilitate individual meetings. However, I always tried very hard not to let go of those sessions. It's always relevant to talk about family of origin issues, and still more so with couples. How your clients learned to handle conflict, how affection was demonstrated within the family, what values they developed from observing their parents' relationship – the answers to these questions may tell you a lot of what you need to know about why your couple is currently at war with one another.

There's one caveat to successful individual sessions: make sure at the start of these meetings that you agree with your client that this is not about learning and keeping secrets from their partner. Keeping secrets as a couple therapist is not a good idea (Silverstein, 1998). Obviously, this doesn't pertain to secrets that aren't directly relevant to the focus of couple therapy or to secrets that may eventually come out but need to be done slowly and carefully, for example, childhood experiences of abuse. But you don't want to find out half-way through your individual session that one person has a secret family two towns over and this is why they are so unavailable to their partner. Ditto secret substance use, infidelity, debt, or anything else that will destroy your alliance with the other half of the couple should it come out that you knew this all along and kept it to yourself. I generally issue this warning in front of both people at the end of the first session, and then reiterate it at the start of the individual sessions so that no one has any concerns about the possibility of secret-keeping.

To provide fair and balanced coverage to this issue, I did once read an academic article that suggested it was no big deal for therapists to keep infidelity secret even as the therapist worked towards improving the relationship for the couple presenting for therapy. I think the author was French, which I suspect was quite relevant to their philosophical positioning on the question and one of those diversity-related issues we'll address further in Chapter 10.

Establishing goals – always important, now super-duper important

Agreement on goals between clients and clinicians is one of the main common factors associated with improvement in therapy (Norcross, 2002; Norcross & Hill, 2004), and I am a strong believer when it comes to doing so with individuals. In couple therapy, the importance of setting goals gets cranked up to 11 out of 10, not unlike the band's speakers in the movie *Spinal Tap*. The increased salience in goals when you're working with couples is because each member of the couple might have different and sometimes conflicting goals: one person may be determined to save the relationship at all costs while the other person may have already decided that splitting up is their preferred outcome. One partner may be dead-set on having children while the other person is equally determined not to. One person wants to retire, buy a boat, and sail around the world, the other person has had literal nightmares about such an experience. In some cases, there is absolutely no middle ground to be identified, but keep in mind that it's not your job to decide which set of goals is more suitable for that couple. Your job is much harder: to help them figure out what matters more to them in life – their relationship or this issue causing the logjam.

Be especially wary when setting goals in couple therapy of mushy, unclear language. For example, when one or both members of a couple tells me that they'd like to work on "communication," I've come to understand that, often, what they really mean is some version of the following: "If you teach me better communication skills, I will be able to more persuasively explain my side of the conflict, and my partner will then be forced to accept that my version of reality is the correct one. We will then implement my preferred solution." Of course, the real issue is that both people feel their position is the most correct one, and they just need the right words to get that across to the person on the other side of the couch. For me, the most helpful response at this juncture would be to push one or ideally both people to spell out exactly what they hope better communication would accomplish – what would stop, what would start, and what would change. This is generally a much greater help in getting to the heart of the issue than "improved communication."

As you do this work, don't think that the main metric for your success as a couple therapist is whether or not the couples who present for therapy ultimately decide to stay together. Sometimes the right answer for both people really is that the relationship comes to an end, calmly, and for the right reasons. Your job then is to help the pair in your room accomplish that with as much empathy and respect for one another as possible. Helping people to process the grief of a relationship breakup can also be very meaningful work even if it's not a classically fairytale ending (most fairytales don't include therapists in any case).

You don't need to be in the perfect relationship to do this work

In her self-help book/memoir *I Didn't Sign Up for This* (2023), couple therapist Dr. Tracy Dalgleish tells the story of a client who spotted her and her husband out in public at a farmer's market looking in every respect like the perfect, affectionate couple. The next session, the client explained that some of Tracy's recommendations were difficult to implement because unlike her therapist, she *didn't* have an amazing marriage. This was an especially poignant moment as throughout the book, Dr. Dalgleish detailed her own struggles with the complexities of being in a long-term relationship while also raising two children and managing a successful business. To be completely fair to her husband, I am 100% on his side on whether it's okay to leave banana peels in the sink (it is not).

If you find yourself entering the field of couple therapy and your own relationship isn't amazing or even amazing-adjacent, please don't feel like an impostor or that you can't do this kind of work. If you have long-standing conflicts, if your arguments sometimes get heated, if you often end up slumped on the couch together rewatching old *Futurama* episodes instead of holding hands and discussing your personal "dream board" for the relationship, you can still be of help to your clients. If anything, your personal experience may give you a better understanding of the nuance and complexity of relationship problems. You'll know in a completely visceral way that the couple arguing about how to spend weekends, how to negotiate custody with an ex-partner, or how to spend money isn't going to resolve these issues in a few weeks, and you can help shape their expectations appropriately. They're climbing their own mountain; even if you yourself are also climbing a mountain, you can still look over across the range and suggest a different route to them, even as you ponder the best route for yourself (Hayes et al., 1999).

On the flip side, you may gain a greater appreciation for your own relationship through doing this work. By the time I started doing couple therapy, I had been with my partner for almost 15 years, and often drove into work gnashing my teeth over arguments related to work hours or chores or any of the other longstanding issues that inevitably build up when you spend that kind of time with another human. However, a couple of sessions with couples sharing stories of infidelity or soul-destroying five-hour arguments, or in-laws who randomly show up at the house to rearrange the kitchen often left me singing a different tune as I left the office, or at least until I saw the state of the kitchen garbage when I got home (my husband likes to play "garbage chicken" – whoever caves and takes out the garbage first is the chicken and has therefore lost).

If you're not in a relationship, that's fine too. As therapists, we are often called upon to work with people with whom we have little or no shared experience (see Chapter 10) and our outsider's perspective can still be extremely useful. Before I had a child myself, I worked with a lot of clients who had children; now that I have a child, I have a different perspective, but it's not automatically a better perspective, just a different one. Your role as a couple therapist is to rise above the day-to-day arguments to see the conflict play out on a larger scale across time, to identify recurring patterns and dysfunctional responses, to help both people make different choices and rebuild trust and intimacy. You don't need to be in your own relationship to do that, and you might even have a more useful perspective as someone not embedded in those conflicts yourself. For example, you won't have lingering resentment over having recently lost "garbage chicken."

Healing long-broken bones

Motivation is often a challenge in therapy: many individual clients have just enough energy to make an appointment for therapy and get themselves through the door of the office before collapsing on the couch. I think many cherish a secret fantasy that they can hand the therapist a jumbled Rubik's cube of their pain, who will then lovingly unscramble it and hand it back to them. Unfortunately, my emotional Rubik's cube unscrambler has been in the shop for some time now and clients instead have to do the work themselves in the face of significant inertia and strong emotions pushing them to keep things the way they've always been. However, at least they are in complete control of the change process.

In couple therapy, issues of motivation are compounded. Research shows that the interval between the development of a problem and entering couple therapy is often two-three years (Doherty et al., 2021). Imagine, if you will, a person showing up to a physician's office with a leg they broke two-three years ago. There's not only the original damage to the bone that needs to be addressed, there's also the collateral damage that occurred in the intervening years, which may actually be worse than the original injury. This is a fundamental truth of couple therapy: the main damage to the relationship is often not the content of the conflict but the process by which the couple has attempted to address it. In other words, it's not the overflowing kitchen garbage *per se*, it's what one partner said to the other about the overflowing kitchen garbage and how the other person responded.

A common situation that I encountered in couple work was for one half of the couple to spend weeks – if not months – begging the other to go to therapy to address their issues. Finally, in the heat of the 18th argument about the issue, the reluctant partner would shout, "Fine! I'll go to therapy if it will shut you up!!" I would then see them a week later, when this momentary flicker of motivation had faded, and the reluctant partner was once again firmly entrenched in their belief that couple therapy was useless and a waste of time. It was a comparatively rare occurrence to see two people with the same level of motivation at the same time, eager to sit down and individually take responsibility for their part in the cycle of conflict (as I write this, I'm picturing a pair of enthusiastic golden retrievers). Discrepancies in motivation may then continue throughout therapy. One person might work up the courage to soften their approach, only to get bitten in response by a partner who's not yet in the same headspace, causing the first person to throw up their hands and report, "I tried but they just reacted the way they always do! There's just no point." Couples can be like magnets: you succeed in convincing one of them to stop doing their usual, problematic behaviour and the other one pulls them right back in.

More so than individual therapy, you, the therapist, need to give yourself grace. You need to give yourself, and the couple, permission to take small steps. You need to help them set realistic expectations of what progress is going to look like and how long it might take, as well as normalize setbacks and barriers to progress. They will need lots of space and time to experiment with new ways of being to find the same wavelength at the same moment. Keep in mind that there is a flip side to vicious cycles of conflict: virtuous cycles are also possible. Couples who want to make their relationships work are often desperate to find a way back to one another. A small act of kindness, a tender softening, an honest conversation can pay dividends if both people have the courage to shift themselves out of dysfunctional patterns.

The balancing act

One of the misconceptions that a lot of clients have about couple therapy is that the therapist is there to take sides or to be judge and jury, to figure out who's right in the conflict and then to champion that person. This mistake assumption might go a long way to explaining why they also don't want to pay $250 an hour to have someone chime in "Yeah!!" for every criticism their partner has been making about them for the past decade.

As you know, that is not your role. Your client is neither of the partners – it is the relationship itself (Doss et al., 2005; Gottlieb et al., 2008). In the tennis game of marriage, you're not a coach for one person or the other but more like a referee: you sit on the really high chair and watch them lob the ball back and forth at each other to get a feel for the pattern of their conflict. You're not on anyone's side: in fact, if you do your job properly, both people are likely to be annoyed at you because you'll be pointing out how both are contributing to the problem. This is why sports referees and couple therapists are so beloved in our society.

To be an effective couple therapist, you need to be very good at multitasking, even more so than with individual therapy. While one person is talking about a painful memory or frustrating interaction, you need to be listening to their words, trying to fit that story into the historical context of the relationship, noting the talking partner's non-verbals, paying attention to the non-verbals of the listening partner, and keeping an eye on the reactions of the talking partner to the listening partner's non-verbals (phew, it was a lot just typing that out!). An eyebrow raise, a nose wrinkle, or the hint of a sneer can send your session from 0 to 60 miles per hour in five seconds. This, not surprisingly, takes a lot of practice over time as well as a lot of day-to-day energy. You need to be alert for misplaced tennis balls of conflict flying towards your face.

Couple therapy countertransference

You've probably experienced some feelings of countertransference feelings in individual psychotherapy: the person sitting across from you reminds you of your racist ex-boss and there's nothing you'd like more than to crush his head like a grape, but you can't because you're a professional (also, it's assault). This feeling gets dialed up even further with couple work because, as I've been saying, everything in couple therapy is stronger and more powerful. If you are a person who has ever been in a dating or romantic relationship, the odds are quite good that someday a couple will walk into your office and describe a situation that feels eerily familiar (Kaslow, 2001). Maybe you are also in a relationship with someone who can't put their phone down long enough to listen to you talk about your day. Maybe you also have a meddling mother-in-law who has made a disparaging remark about every child-rearing decision you've made from the moment of conception onwards. Maybe your partner also puts the dishes right-next-to-but-not-actually-in the dishwasher, even though it would take the exact same amount of energy to just do it properly, geez. Note that this experience is different from the values talk we had earlier. Values within couple therapy refer to the larger perspective on the ideal resolution for various kinds of conflict, whereas countertransference refers to that in-the-moment tidal wave of rage that might come for you if one of your clients happens to roll their eyes in the exact same way your loving partner does when you ask whether he's golfing again this weekend too.

In that moment of realizing that the conflict being discussed in the room is a blast from your past, or even your present, your lizard brain will probably try to hijack your cortex and help you see that this is a wonderful opportunity to set the offending client right, in the way you haven't been able to do with your own partner. Resist the urge. Notice it, take a breath. Stare at your office plant for a few seconds to reset your brain. Visualize putting that urge in a filing cabinet labelled "my own stuff" that you can unlock and deal with when your day is done. If you haven't already done so, consider couple therapy for yourself or maybe read a book or two with a focus on improving or processing your own situation. But whatever you do, don't take sides, no matter how stupid that dishes-next-to-the-dishwasher behaviour truly is.

Healing from infidelity, or why couples should discuss whether or not sexting with other people is okay

The years I did couple therapy were marked by a veritable epidemic of "sexters" and the people they had wronged. In fact, I would estimate that 80–90% of my infidelity cases involved only virtual contact, which the sexters argued "didn't count," though their partners saw it otherwise. To be fair, it's not altogether surprising that people don't agree on whether sexting is cheating given that most people can't even agree on what "counts" as sex (Byers et al., 2009). However, the feelings of betrayal and broken trust were often just as substantial for the virtual cheating as they were for cheating involving human contact (Drouin et al., 2017; Falconer & Humphreys, 2019; Klettke et al., 2014).

When it comes to infidelity, don't always feel you need to look for deeper motivations or dysfunctional early life experiences. Over the long term, day-to-day relationships can get monotonous – there are bills to pay, chores to do, obligatory trips to family weddings that are cash bar only. On the other hand, cheating is fun. There are no obligations, no baggage, no chores, just the sexy part of relationships with a bunch of exciting, dirty secrets and sneaking around. Yikes, I'm really selling cheating here! The point is, sometimes people cheat because their pappy cheated and their grandpappy cheated and their great-grandpappy cheated (maybe he mailed dirty daguerrotypes?) and they learned that the fidelity part of the marriage vows is optional. But sometimes they cheat because adult life can be boring and mundane and cheating is idealized as the antidote.

If you are currently in a monogamous romantic partnership, please put this book down and go have a conversation with your partner right now about whether or not sexting constitutes cheating. Be very clear, and very specific, possibly using examples about where you stand on nude pictures, mild flirtation, and saucy conversation. And then – this is crucial – abide by those rules.

The magic that keeps couples together

Doing couple therapy gave me a renewed appreciation for my own long-term relationship. After a full day of hearing about the challenges of blending families or learning to trust again after infidelity, it was often easier to put the problems of my own marriage in perspective and to find more goodwill for my husband and his annoying dishwasher issues. You may be surprised and inspired by the problems that couples can overcome together. I've often heard friends and family say, "If my spouse ever cheated/hid debt from me/trashed a hotel room in a drunken rage, I'd never forgive them" but I saw people forgive each other for all those things and more. This kind of therapy work is hard, harder even than individual therapy, but I've seen people show up despite the pain and heartache to do the work because nothing matters more to them than their partnership. As a long-time couple therapist said to me early in my career, we never truly understand the magic that keeps a couple together. A certain level of humility and appreciation for mystery is required to do this work.

Conclusion

Our romantic relationships are central to many of our identities, often one of the most important and meaningful connections of our entire lives (Apostolou et al., 2023; Braithwaite & Holt-Lunstad, 2017); it is unsurprising, therefore, that problems in this area can represent one of life's major stressors (Chait Barnett et al., 2005; Snyder & Halford, 2012). This is why the stakes are so high, this is why the arguments can be so vicious, this is why the despair is so palpable. But if you pursue couple therapy, you have a chance to help people untangle themselves from this knotted mess in which they find themselves, and that can be deeply meaningful work. Find a way to remind yourself of this often.

Chapter 9

Inpatient settings

If your work preferences are for variety, a fast pace, and lots of problem-solving, you will probably enjoy working with patients in hospital settings. You'll get to see a breadth of presenting issues in a fascinating cross-section of patients, working with complex and severe cases. Hospital jobs or training placements offer a real chance to live the ethos of biopsychosocial work, taking a holistic perspective on physical and mental health and wellness as part of a multidisciplinary team composed of psychiatry, medicine, nursing, physiotherapy, occupational therapy, pharmacy, and other fascinating specialties. Not only that, but it's also your opportunity to feel like a cast member on *Grey's Anatomy*! All that being said, the challenge of treating cases with severe symptoms alongside a group of people who may or may not understand the work you do (and vice versa) can be intense and sometimes overwhelming, and a few pointers might be helpful.[1]

Introduction to multidisciplinary teams

Working on multidisciplinary teams gives you an unparalleled ability to provide comprehensive, wraparound care to patients and their families. It's also a wonderful chance to step on people's toes and occasionally crash into one another, like dancers performing a ballet together with no rehearsal. It would be lovely if the multiday orientation sessions that are usually required to start work at hospitals involved various representatives from the different professions introducing themselves and explaining their scope of practice. Sadly, this has never been my experience. Instead, the presentations usually focused more on the hospital's vision statement,

---

1 Note that in this one chapter, I will use the term "patients" rather than "clients" as this is more typical language use in these types of settings.

DOI: 10.4324/9781003355366-12

inspirational speeches from lesser vice presidents, and whether you should go into a room with a big orange sign saying "biohazard area" (usually no).

Hospitals are usually fast-paced and constantly on the verge of chaos, now more than ever. If there are few formal opportunities for learning and no one has time to grab lunch and explain what it is they do around here, how do you figure it out? Here's a few strategies:

- Attend multidisciplinary meetings, whenever possible. A good opportunity for this is going to patient rounds, which might involve one person presenting a case to an audience drawn from around the hospital, a small team standing in a semi-circle in a hallway moving from room to room, or a group sitting around a boardroom discussing the list of recent admissions. Listen and pay attention to what role everyone plays in patient care. Rounds are also a great chance to learn about other neat things like what diet is best for patients recovering from severe burns and how many people get injured doing home repairs while drunk (answer: so, so many).
- Grab a few minutes to chat whenever you can. If the physiotherapist is coming into the patient's room as you are leaving, ask them what they are focusing on in their meeting today, which will also help you in your work with the patient. If the people at the nursing station aren't frantically busy (a rare occurrence), you can take a few minutes to ask them the difference between a charge nurse and a floor nurse, or how practice differs between the intensive care and the med-surg units.
- Socialize outside of work, if possible. After-work gatherings are a great way to find out more about the different specialties, or at least, what things annoy them about working in this hospital.

Most healthcare professionals involved in mental health have a wide scope of practice so the specific tasks assigned to psychology, psychiatry, social work, nursing, occupational therapy, or pastoral care at any given hospital may vary quite a bit (Ashcroft et al., 2019; Talmi et al., 2016). For example, if you've worked at a hospital where social workers deliver psychotherapy, it's a little disorienting if they specialize in discharge-planning in another setting. Sometimes therapy groups are the exclusive province of psychology and sometimes you'll find mental health nurses doing most of the facilitation. At every new placement, you'll need to learn the unique responsibilities of the different groups in that setting, recognizing also that some of these decisions about who does what and why may be the dust-covered legacy of choices originally made decades ago by people who are no longer around to explain their logic.

As you get up to speed at a new hospital, think of yourself as a curious anthropologist, observing the social structure of its denizens, like Jane

Goodall and the chimpanzees (just don't refer to your colleagues as monkeys no matter how apt they may be to fling poop). Listen, watch, pay attention, ask questions if someone stops moving long enough, and have patience with everyone, especially yourself.

Handling disagreements

In recent years, other healthcare professionals are getting more training in mental health (Booth et al., 2017; Caulfield et al., 2019). Broadly speaking, this is a step in the right direction: more mental health literacy and attention to the bidirectional relationship between mental and physical health are necessary for effective patient care. However, learning just a bit about mental health is a wonderful example of that idiom, "Knowing enough to be dangerous." I do think that greater awareness of mental health issues among non-mental health specialties has directly contributed to some very awkward moments in my career, like the time a surgeon stood next to me and incorrectly listed the symptoms of schizophrenia to a group of surgical residents.

I've been asked about handling conflict or resolving ethical challenges on multidisciplinary teams in pretty much every job interview I've ever attended. The short answer is that you address these concerns on a multidisciplinary team exactly the way you'd address them on any other team: you act like a reasonable, polite, respectful human being, trusting that disagreements and conflict are largely the result of miscommunication or misunderstanding rather than sheer assholery, until proven otherwise (Brown et al., 2011).

Sometimes you're going to find yourself in a situation where another team member has given some incorrect psychoeducation to a patient about a mental health issue or made recommendations that range from ineffective to straight-up contraindicated. If you catch this error in a note in someone's chart, it's easy enough to make a correction to the patient verbally: "I noticed that Dr. So-and-so suggested you try (incorrect advice) but actually more recent research suggests (correct advice). Let's try (correct advice) first and I'll put that in my note so they can see I've made this recommendation." If another team member gives incorrect guidance in front of you, the issue becomes trickier, depending on the personalities involved; in this situation, being a student or relatively early in your career may actually work to your advantage. Start by validating anything at all the other person has said that is correct – "Yes, PTSD is certainly a potential diagnosis to consider here" – and then politely, respectfully explain that more recent evidence that you learned in your coursework supports an alternative explanation or approach with this problem – "But current research does not support making any kind of mental health diagnosis if the patient is in a medically-induced coma and unable to actively partici-pate in the assessment." Yes, this was a completely true example and, for the record, it's not really possible to diagnose anything in the DSM if the patient is unconscious.

There may occasionally be moments where for ethical reasons, you are pushed to flat out contradict another specialty, either to their face or to a third party. In one setting, I had to go directly to a patient's physician and explain that under no circumstances should an extremely suicidal person with easy access to a gun be discharged, despite what other professionals might have said about their stability and wellbeing. There's always time to smooth things over later and it's better to have a psychiatrist give you dirty looks every time they see you than to have a patient's death on your conscience.

Working on multidisciplinary teams will give you a marvelous chance to develop your professional assertiveness and communication skills. Or at least it'll give you a lot to talk about when you inevitably get that "conflict resolution" question at an interview.

Take the information in patients' charts with a grain of salt

Depending on their history, some patients may be admitted with several volumes of paperwork about them, including notes and reports on pre-vious assessments and treatments, diagnoses considered and ruled in/out, and accounts of interactions with staff members. Much of this documen-tation may be helpful to you as you plan what further data to gather and what treatments might be relevant for your patient. However, these notes may also be characterized by prejudiced comments and non-evidence-based speculation about the "meaning" of the patient's presentation and behaviours. For example, at one hospital, the psychiatrists routinely diagnosed patients with dyed hair, piercings, and tattoos as "attention-seeking," which was met with a lot of eyerolls from the hair-dyed, pierced, and tattooed staff at our clinic.

Your choice of what to do with the information from a patient's chart can be a surprisingly controversial issue in psychotherapy. Some therapists suggest that you don't look at it at all: come to the patient as a blank slate, ready to hear their story fresh and untainted by previous perspectives. Others say to read every document you can get your hands on so that you're better prepared and don't waste your time or the patient's. Patients themselves may prefer that you not read the chart if they've had a lot of negative interactions with staff that they are concerned were documented unfairly. Or they may strongly prefer that you do read their chart because they don't want to repeat a bunch of tedious information that you could easily look up yourself.

Here's my recommendation: if you can, ask the patient first. Patients don't have a lot of autonomy in hospital settings and it's always nice when we can give them some back. If a manager or supervisor requires you to read some or all of the document, let them know that you are going to do it before you do so. No one likes to meet someone for the first time and hear, "Nice to meet you! My name is Dr. Ménard and I just read a binder full of information about your history of substance use, your relationships with family members, and your bowel habits." When you do read it, focus on the most relevant and recent sections of the chart, taking previous accounts with a grain of salt, and follow up with the patient where there may be areas of potential controversy or disagreement. And no matter what you may hear from other health professionals at your hospital, simply having tattoos is not an indicator of anything other than an interest in having tattoos.

Advocating for patients

One of the aspects that I most enjoyed about hospital work was being able to spend more time with patients compared to other healthcare specialties. Patient meetings in hospitals were usually far shorter than the usual 50-minute outpatient session that characterize psychotherapy but generally quite a bit longer than a typical interaction with a medical specialist. Physicians, residents, and nurses have heavy caseloads and little extra time to spend in relationship-building chit-chat (Irving et al., 2017; Linzer et al., 2016); in contrast, I was often able to pull up a chair – literally and figuratively – to get to know patients. This allowed me the opportunity to learn valuable details about their lives, providing much-needed context for the issues that might interact with their physical problems and helping me advocate for them with their team, who might not have understood the complex factors driving their behaviour.

Mental health professionals in hospitals are often called on by medical teams to figure out why a patient won't "comply"[2] with a treatment regime, the implication being that we should subtly or unsubtly push them to just cooperate, dammit. In one instance, a patient was stating that they would not be taking time off post-surgery despite medical orders to do so. Their treatment team was understandably aggravated that the patient would risk worsening the injury, requiring readmission and further interventions. After one meeting with the patient, my student found out that

2 I *strongly* recommend that you push back wherever and whenever you hear the word "comply," which is a demeaning term and should never be used by anyone in healthcare. Like the Rolling Stones, this word is long overdue for retirement.

they were the sole provider for their children, had no medical leave or short-term disability from their job that could cover the financial shortfall of taking time off, and had no supportive friends or family able or willing to help: a week or more of medical leave would mean the whole family might get evicted and/or go hungry. We used this information to collaborate with the rest of the team on a plan to minimize the risk of compromising their recent treatment while also ensuring the ongoing health and safety of their family. Solutions in these cases may involve finding the compromise options in their medical care or connecting the patient with much-needed community resources and trouble-shooting their ability to access those resources.

Spending time with and advocating for patients and their families when they are in pain, scared, or vulnerable is an enormous privilege of working in hospitals. Your efforts in this area can lead to smoother, more effective care for the patient and their families, as well as smoother, happier functioning of multidisciplinary teams. It's win-win, baby!

Losing patients

Depending on the population you see and the settings where you work, you may experience the deaths of patients in your care. I was taught in graduate school that up to a quarter of clinical psychologists at some point in their career will lose a client to suicide (Chemtob et al., 1988; Finlayson & Graetz Simmonds, 2018), but unfortunately, the lecture stopped there. None of my classes addressed losing patients to illness or injury in other settings or, crucially, how to manage that very specific kind of grief. This was a serious omission given how deeply mental health professionals may be affected by the loss of their patients (Darden & Rutter, 2011; Finlayson & Graetz Simmonds, 2018).

During my time in hospital settings, I did lose a few patients to natural causes; in some cases, the death was quite foreseeable due to grave illness or injury, while in other cases, it was a surprise even to the rest of the treatment team. I saw one patient come in with an aortic dissection, a condition normally known for being highly fatal, who had been rescued by a friend unexpectedly stopping by their house at the perfect moment to call an ambulance. During our brief meetings, the patient talked about what a lucky break this had been and how they were going to use this miracle to galvanize some health-related changes in their life. Unfortunately, they died quite suddenly and the lucky break they described seemed like nothing more than a cruel joke by the universe. On another occasion, the patient had fallen into a coma following an overdose; their partner, who described their own struggles with sobriety, kept repeating that any level of functioning in the patient would be acceptable as long as they were still alive. But the patient died, and I never saw the partner again despite my encouragement to pursue outpatient psychotherapy.

There are a lot of different reasons that a patient's death might touch you. You might have spent quite a bit of time with them and their families and come to care deeply for them. You might have a medical condition in common with them and this may push you to empathize more strongly. They might share demographic characteristics with friends or family members and their loss reminds you of the inevitability of losing your own loved ones. The loss of a patient for any reason is difficult, and there are lots of factors that can affect your response. If it happens to you or to a student under your supervision, I suggest that you take some time to process, either with other mental health professionals or with other professionals from their care team who might also have had a connection to the patient. Try to focus on the support and care you provided in their last few days or weeks and how that may have helped them to worry less, cope better, or feel some sense of calm.

Repeat yourself

"I gotta go, a nurse just came in." I can't tell you how many times I heard these words as I walked into a room and a patient ended a phone call. This despite the fact that my opening line with everyone was always some version of "Hi, I'm Dr. Ménard. I'm a psychologist here at the hospital and your team asked me to come see you."

Patients meet a lot of different people in a very short span of time when they are admitted to hospital, and some of them are better at introducing themselves than others. Many different healthcare professions also dress alike, in scrubs or a white coat, so that's often not helpful in making distinctions between different providers. Also – and I can't emphasize this enough – people admitted to hospital are often not thinking very clearly due to physical pain, anxiety about their illness or injury, massive changes in sleep and eating, loneliness, concerns about their jobs or finances or loved ones, and just plain garden-variety stress. Deeply stressed-out people are not the best at taking in, retaining, or recalling information of any kind (Schwabe & Wolf, 2010; Twomey et al., 2020).

What all of this means is that you will need to repeat yourself a lot, way more than you might normally do in clinical practice. This is true for your name and function in the hospital, any recommendations you have for the patient, the next time you will meet with them, and any other valuable and relevant information. Have the patient write a note or put it in their phone; if a family member is handy, give them this information too. Your guiding principle for the correct amount of repetition is "just short of annoying the patient."

There will be smells

There's no getting around it, if you work in a hospital: there are going to be unpleasant smells in your work life. At best, hospitals tend to smell like institutional-grade disinfectant, which is not usually ranked highly on anyone's list of favourite odours. At worst, noxious smells you may encounter in these settings include bodily fluids of various types, badly infected wounds, unwashed bodies, and topical medications; more often than not, it's a mix of everything on the previous list. Unfortunately, there's not much problem-solving to be done about most of these issues. Patients may need to wait for assistance to shower and groom themselves and believe me, they are no happier about delays in their hygiene activities than you are. Wearing face masks does serve a dual role as infection control and smell-barrier so that might be one good option. Another option might be to spritz a handkerchief (check your grandmother's sock drawer) with a perfume or essential oil that you enjoy and leave that in your pocket as an antidote to bring to your nose as needed. The good news is that I caught colds and flus much more frequently when I worked in hospital settings, so my nose was often blocked and smell was a moot point (okay, maybe more mixed news).

Thinking on your feet

When you're working in hospital settings, you may find yourself confronted with a problem you have never previously encountered or a limitation to therapy you hadn't envisaged during training. Depending on the availability of relevant clinical or research literature, you may be called on to improvise in creative ways (Sheaves et al., 2018; Tafrate et al., 2014). For example, consider that most behavioural activation interventions (e.g., cooking dinner, doing a hobby) require that the patient has some freedom and autonomy to choose their daily activities as well as access to the necessary equipment. Progressive muscle relaxation may be challenging for people who are not in complete control of their limbs. When I worked in a prison, my mother thought it might be a nice group therapy intervention to teach the prisoners to knit, so that they'd have a practical and enjoyable hobby. She didn't understand that "sharps" of most types are carefully controlled in such settings, especially with people who have a documented history of stabbing one another. You'll need to learn how to take the basic principles of the interventions you've learned and look for ways to make them happen under limited circumstances, which is not a bad thing for the patients to learn either.

This creative improvisation may extend even to the delivery of therapy itself. On one occasion, I was asked to see a patient who had recently received serious spinal cord injuries and had been left paralyzed from the neck down. We sometimes saw non-verbal patients at the hospital but for this work, we generally relied on writing or a letter board where patients could point and spell out their thoughts. I asked the nurses what they expected me to do in this situation where the patient couldn't speak or spell and they said they didn't know but they couldn't stand to see the person lying in bed with tears streaming down their face. Fair enough. In this instance, we managed to communicate through a combination of head nods and shakes; I tried to address a broad range of stressors with yes/no questions and organize my follow-up questions like the branching of a tree, making sure to following a concern through to its most specific details before returning to other potential issues in the same group and then to other types of stressors. For example: are you worried about your family? Nod. Are you worried about your mother? Nod. Are you worried about her stress? Nod. Are you worried she's not taking care of herself while you're here in the hospital? Shake. Are you worried about her being able to go to work? Shake. Do you worry that she needs to spend more time with your younger siblings? Nod. Would you like us to try to share this with her when she gets here? Nod. Let's get back to other family members: are you worried about your brother? Although cumbersome and time-consuming, this style of intervention was surprisingly effective. In particular, this patient, who was in their early 20s, had been worried about their ability to have children after the accident; I was able to relay this concern to their medical team so that their physicians could have a more in-depth conversation of what might or might not be possible down the road.

Working in hospitals means learning how to quickly and effectively search the literature for evidence-based clues and strategies to address your patients' concerns, but it also means adapting the principles you know to be effective for other issues as best you can. While it may feel frustrating to offer interventions that have less-than-solid support, try to keep in mind that some genuine and patient-centred help, however flawed and incomplete, is generally better than nothing at all when caring for worried patients.

Doing therapy in inhospitable spaces

It would be lovely if hospitals had therapy rooms set up on every floor, with comfortable chairs, throw pillows, soft but unobtrusive lighting, a plant in the corner, calming paintings, maybe a coffee machine or water cooler... a gal can dream. Unfortunately, that is rarely the case; more often than not, you'll find yourself doing therapy in a conference room, at the patient's bedside or in a space that suspiciously resembles a utility closet (buckets, mops, and cleaning supplies are usually a dead giveaway).

Do what you can with what you've got. If you're using a conference room, check with the nurses before your meeting with the patient to see if an entire troupe of physicians is going to march into the room 5 minutes into your session and demand the space. In my experience, some professions are more responsive to pushback and negotiation than others, but I wouldn't try your luck with psychiatrists – I didn't win many battles with them. In hospital ward-style rooms where you can't guarantee that you won't be overheard, highlight that for the patient and ask if they still want to talk. If you're at a patient's bedside, ask visiting family members to leave so that the patient can speak openly: for example, "I hear the cafeteria has lovely coffee," even if you know that's an egregious lie (which it always is in hospitals). If your therapy room doubles as a utility closet, make sure the mops in the corner of the room are contained so that they don't come crashing down in the middle of a session or better yet, hide them behind the broken filing cabinet you're sure to find in there as well. When all else fails, make a joke or comment about the situation. Patients can tolerate a lot of odd set-ups if you're trying to help them, but I find it's much smoother when we mutually agree that the setting is less-than-desirable rather than try to pretend that coatrooms are a normal space for a group therapy session.

Hold your expectations lightly

Inpatients on a psychiatric unit have often experienced a whole world of treatment prior to meeting you for the first time: every medication under the sun, every therapy with a three-letter acronym as its name, short- or long-term stints in rehab, alternative therapies, and/or electroconvulsive therapy. As a new therapist, I often felt very daunted seeing such patients: what could I possibly bring to the table that was new or helpful? Here's a mantra for these moments: don't assume you will make a difference and don't assume that you won't.

On one occasion, I was asked to see a patient on the inpatient psychiatric unit who was known for having a "chip on their shoulder" and as a result, was frequently in conflict with other patients and with staff members. They had already seen many other professionals in that setting and took a dim view of being asked to see yet another "useless shrink" (their words). I wouldn't describe our psychotherapy sessions as smooth sailing but eventually, we made some tangible progress and the patient was noticeably less irritable and snappy. As we prepared to wrap up, I asked the patient what they thought about our work together and they gave me the following compliment: "It wasn't as big a waste of time as I thought it was going to be." Music to my ears, dear reader. Remember those types of comments and relish them during the hard times.

Sometimes, you may be the clinician who arrives on the spot at the exact right moment to support a patient as they put learning into action because their circumstances have changed enough to finally allow it. The 14th medication that they've tried may actually be the one that gives them the energy they needed to implement some strategies that will make a difference in their life. You may bring up just the right idea at just the right moment for the patient to really hear it properly for the first time, even if three other clinicians brought it up before you. When people are ready to hear something, they can pick it up just about anywhere. Note that this goes both ways: I can't tell you how many people I had been working with for months ascribe their sudden understanding and change to a segment they had recently seen on *Oprah*.

You may also find yourself being the right therapist at the wrong moment in someone's life. A patient's treatment for anxiety is going along swimmingly until their spouse suddenly announces they want a divorce and leaves the next day. A patient's treatment for depression is unexpectedly compromised by a child's diagnosis with cancer, their life's priorities rearranged overnight. Relationship endings, deaths, job loss, sudden illnesses or injuries, financial crises – life's catastrophes have no respect for your carefully thought-out treatment plan. There are so many factors that can influence someone's mental health that it's almost inevitable that you will sometimes end up on the losing side due to uncontrollable external circumstances. Unfortunately for you and the patient, these things happen.

Don't beat yourself up if you don't see an obvious change with someone during your work. Your role in a patient's life may simply be to plant the seeds that blossom later. Even if the net result of your interaction was that they believe that there are professionals out there who care about them and are invested in their improvement, that's an excellent legacy to leave.

Disinfect early, disinfect often

When I look back at the periods of my life when I had the greatest number of colds and flus, they often coincided with those times when I was working in a hospital. There's a reason that you find hand sanitizer dispensers attached to the wall every 20 feet in these buildings: they are *crawling* with bacteria and viruses. You might think this germ soup is caused by the sick patients themselves, and they are probably partially to blame, but illnesses in these settings are often spread also by their loving family members and friends, who shrug aside their nagging coughs, their upset stomachs, and their clogged sinuses to come in and visit. Note: if your loved one is in the hospital and you have the sniffles, do a video call instead, I'm begging you.

As a mental healthcare professional in these settings, do what you can to be part of the solution, not part of the problem: sanitize your hands often, wear a mask, and stay home if you're sick (see also Chapter 5 on self-care). And if you hear someone hacking up a lung from the chair next to your patient's bed, maybe come back later, with a can of disinfectant spray in tow.

Don't ascribe to malice what can be satisfactorily explained by boredom

I worry occasionally that healthcare professionals, including the folks who specialize in mental health, can sometimes lose sight of contextual influences on patients' reasons for engaging in problem behaviours. This may result in them digging for deep-seated, complex explanations for challenges that have a much simpler cause. This lesson is especially relevant for work in hospital settings, which are typically noisy, smelly, boring, and generally unpleasant; most patients don't particularly enjoy being there and their behaviour often reflects that mindset. Here are some examples of patient-related difficulties I encountered and the strange theories that members of their healthcare team advanced:

- Why isn't the patient eating? Do they have an eating disorder? Is their lack of appetite indicative of depression? Are visiting family members behaving abusively by taking food from their tray? No! Hospital food is often tasteless and patients don't like it, especially if they are used to good food. Now, why visiting family members sometimes helped themselves to untouched meal trays is an entirely different and strange question but those people weren't my patients so their weird palates were none of my concern.
- Why isn't the patient sleeping? Are they anxious? Are they depressed? Do they have a sleeping disorder? No! Hospitals are *extremely* noisy. There are alarms and monitors and flashing, beeping things in every corner of the room. Sometimes there are hospital codes announced over intercom, site-wide. There are other patients snoring, family members tromping down the hallway, and a guy three rooms down who is withdrawing from benzodiapines and has been yelling for 48 hours straight. It's a wonder anyone sleeps in hospitals.
- Why is the patient sitting around their room in their underwear? Are they an exhibitionist? Do they have symptoms of a personality disorder? No! They have become habituated to medical professionals coming into their room every 45 minutes to do assessments and decided

that this was a more efficient approach than putting on and then pulling off their tie-in-the-back robe repeatedly.
- Why are patients on the unit getting into regular conflict with one another? Do they have antisocial personality disorder? Do they have rage issues? Do they have a fundamental deficit in their communication skills? Actually, yes to all three! But they were also really, really, *really* bored. In some institutions, patients may spend months or even years in close quarters with one another and are very likely to get on each others' nerves at least some of the time. Remember the 2020 COVID-19 lockdowns you spent with your loved ones? That level of friction, but on a longer time scale and without Netflix.

Start with the simplest explanations for problem behaviours; once you rule those out, it's fair to look at formal diagnoses and other deeper explanations, but never rule out the obvious without checking.

Hospital data

Hospital work makes it easy to collect rich data about how your patient interacts in interpersonal relationships, including how they relate with family members and other providers. It's one thing for a patient to tell you a story about a negative interaction they had with a boss or fellow employee; it's quite another to witness yourself the role the patient themselves may play in these conflicts. I sometimes had the experience of sitting at a patient's bedside while our conversation was briefly interrupted by a nurse or another member of the treatment team needing to ask the patient something or remind them of an upcoming test or treatment. "Did you see how rude she was to me?!!" the patient would rage, to my utter bafflement. This surprising response might stem from previous negative interactions with the same provider, previous negative experiences with staff in hospitals, or just strong personality issues, but it was definitely useful clinical data.

On one occasion, a teenager was brought into the hospital for a stab wound, having been a (somewhat) innocent bystander during a drug deal gone wrong. As you might expect, the patient was in a lot of pain and fairly miserable when I went to see them. Their worried father was at the bedside and seemingly couldn't help himself from scolding: "I told you that you were hanging out with the wrong crowd! I told you those were bad people!" I have a strong hunch that most parental advice is likely to be poorly received when the child is distracted by the pain of a recent stab wound, not to mention the cognitive dissonance of having been stabbed by people that they had, until recently, considered friends. This brief interaction gave me a lot of information about their parent–child communication outside of the hospital as well. Maybe the father often failed to take his child's perspective or express empathy when imparting life lessons, leading to his very legitimate concerns about the child's safety being ignored. Maybe the teenager often hid their activities or minimized the harm of them, resulting in dad's increased anxiety. Think of how much more useful this interaction was to witness than the father telling me in my office, "My kid doesn't listen to me." For similar reasons, a social worker friend of mine who works in oncology likes to stop by on his patients' first day of chemotherapy to ask how they are thinking and feeling about the new treatment. The answers he gets and the interventions he can then suggest are a lot more accurate compared to patients' predictions beforehand or their recall afterwards.

Working in a hospital may allow you to collect extremely vivid clinical data, as well as give you the chance to intervene in a much more accurate and timely way.

Conclusion

In the current political and economic landscape, jobs in hospital settings for mental health professionals can be more difficult to find and never seem to be enough to meet the need of the patients, but I'm hopeful that this trend will reverse itself in my lifetime. It's a huge privilege to do this kind of work in a hospital setting, to have the opportunity to see and support people during the worst days of their lives. It can be intense and sometimes very challenging work, but you have the chance to help alleviate overwhelming burdens. This is a profoundly rewarding aspect of the job and it can make all the difference between a devastating, completely unmanageable event for the patient and a devastating event where some hope may be possible.

Chapter 10

Diversity

In recent years, issues of equity, diversity, inclusion, and justice (EDIJ) have received significantly more attention in many areas, including the world of psychotherapy (American Psychological Association, 2003; Jones et al., 2013). This is a very, very good thing and long overdue. Many training programs in counselling and therapy have mandatory multicultural skills classes but it's often just the one class. Ideally, the learning and work of effectively supporting clients from diverse groups will continue until the day you retire.

We all need to do this work

Let me be transparent and upfront about the perspective from which I am writing this chapter and the lenses through which I've trained and worked. I am white, able-bodied, heterosexual, cis-gender, and a citizen of Canada; at one point, I could also say that I was young, but it's been quite a while now since a client commented on my apparent youthfulness and I'm learning to live with that fact. Based on this list, you may suspect that I don't really know what it's like to struggle in my day-to-day life because of discrimination related to some facet of my identity and you'd be right. As a result, this is a scary chapter to write because my gut says that I really shouldn't be the one talking about this, that I'm bound to get stuff wrong, and that I will misidentify the important issues or find other ways to put my foot in my mouth. I think these fears are a necessary part of reckoning with diversity more broadly: it's sometimes nerve-wracking but like most scary things associated with clinical training, it's best to confront this and take ownership for your part of this process. If you haven't done so already, look up "*The Wheel of Privilege and Power*" (Duckworth, 2020) and see where you fall in the various categories. This will help you understand where you fit in relation to your clients and where you may need to do more or less work to make effective connections.

DOI: 10.4324/9781003355366-13

Let's be very clear on this issue: the work of EDIJ cannot fall only on marginalized and minoritized people. For one thing, they're as busy as everyone else with their own stuff. In addition, many don't enjoy being made the "go-to" person for any and all matters related to their demographic membership. But the main reason is that moving towards an equitable future will require *a lot* of people to make changes in research, teaching, and clinical practice, so the majority of the work will need to be done by people who are *not* affected by discrimination and forms of colonial, capitalistic, and racial violence in their day-to-day lives. So let's roll up our collective cardigan sleeves and get on with it – we all deserve better.

Avoid making assumptions about identity

As a graduate student, I saw a client who emigrated to Canada from a country torn apart by civil war. She had lost numerous family members to the violence and had survived a devastating physical injury herself before fleeing her home. She had then rebuilt her life from the ground up: learning English, finding work, and figuring out the day-to-day challenges of living in a foreign country, all while parenting four young children with no support from family or friends. This woman had overcome incredible challenges in her life, and I was deeply insecure about how much help I could be to her. My supervisor highlighted the numerous traumas she had faced and suggested that our work together was likely to focus on the many losses she had experienced and the violence she had witnessed; she advised me to read up on PTSD symptoms in refugees, which I dutifully did. After going through the paperwork and the limits of confidentiality with the client, I asked her what brought her to therapy, that classic opening question. Her response to me was: "I am the mother of four girls." She then proceeded to tell me all about the stress she was feeling because of her eldest daughter, who was making troubling life choices, including substance use and friendships with unsavoury characters (or at least unsavoury according to mom). This was ultimately the entire focus of our work together: the stress of parenting, the centrality of her identity as a mother, and the impact of her daughter's choices on her own self-perceptions, i.e., "Have I failed as a mother?"

No matter how marginalized the groups your client belongs to and no matter how many intersecting identities they inhabit, don't make any assumptions about how the challenges associated with their identity might relate to their priorities for therapy. Have all of these possibilities in your mind but be guided by the client, focus on how they frame their problems, and make sure to put factors like race in the larger context (Chang & Berk, 2009). In her life, my client had managed so many challenges related to her identity as an ethnic minority, as disabled, as a refugee, as a non-English speaker but her main concern was about the piece of her identity that she considered most fundamental to who she was – her parenting role.

Keep in mind that clients who are members of marginalized groups may be sick of healthcare professionals assuming this part of their identity is a major contributor to their problems (Hall et al., 2015; Winter et al., 2016). I've had clients push back hard when I asked about the impact of their identity on their concerns – "Are you saying I'm anxious just because I'm bisexual?! – which led to a lot of empathic backpedalling. However, I've also had clients visibly relax and say some version of "Well, I didn't know how to bring it up here, but I do think that racism *is* playing a role in my work problems." Know that if you do get it wrong – and you almost certainly will at some point so go ahead and embrace that inevitability – empathic backpedalling can succeed, especially if you have a good alliance with the client. If your colleagues are willing, consider having them role play getting mad at you so that you can practice your backpedalling. Making a mistake, taking responsibility, and behaving differently going forward can be a powerful, reparative experience for a client in therapy; while minoritized clients may be very used to people in their lives saying ignorant stuff to them, apologizing effectively and changing your behaviour may be a less common and very welcome experience.

Recognize and manage your assumptions

Over the years, I've seen clients from all different backgrounds, who differed in every conceivable dimension from me. I've sometimes had a lot of doubts about whether a client would be interested in working with me because of our differences. My mind kept expecting them to say, "You're just some 25-year-old white girl, what the hell do you know about being an incarcerated Indigenous man/an older Black woman/a gay man with HIV/ a disabled immigrant?" But even if they occasionally thought it – which would be very fair – none of those clients ever articulated such doubts to me out loud, suggesting that they were at least willing to take a chance on me, for which I remain grateful even now. I had incorrectly assumed that clients would reject my support based on our differences.

Conversely, keep an eye out for over-confidence in any situation where you are coming in as an outsider, whether based on ethnicity, socio-economic status, or otherwise. If you're having thoughts along the lines of "All these clients need is…" or "I'm making a difference" or any sentence involving the word "rescue," you may be in danger of falling victim to the Savior complex (often but not always related to being white). If you recognize a thought you've had in that list, don't feel bad – Hollywood has made billions of dollars promoting the idea that all Black inner-city students really need to succeed in life is a Michelle Pfeiffer-type to come and rescue them. But do seek supervision and start building an EDIJ-themed reading list. Keep in mind that the amount of help you can provide your clients will likely fall somewhere between 0 and 100% but probably not too close to either extreme; either way, your clients will always be doing the heavy lifting themselves.

Some clients will highlight identity differences with you the therapist, but it may not always be the differences you'd expect. For example, when I worked in the United States, I saw a lot of older, Black clients from lower SES backgrounds, but I heard very few comments about those differences; however, many of them did highlight the fact that I was obviously Canadian (Oh ya bud, I guess my accent is pretty strong, eh?). At another job, an older male client who was a devout religious believer couldn't believe that I did not share his convictions and brought this up in many sessions. I've had male clients who couldn't talk about their sexual problems because I was female, despite my research expertise in that area (I literally co-authored a book about magnificent sex[1]). So, expect the unexpected when it comes to differences between you and your clients and consider their area of focus to be a valuable source of information about their issues. When in doubt, assess further to discover why this particular identity difference matters to the client and what the discrepancy between you and them means from their perspective.

On the flip side, watch out for situations where you and the client occupy a lot of the same groups, when you or the client might assume a lot of shared experience that may not be accurate. I've worked with a lot of young, white women, some of whom were even studying psychology or mental health, and I can confidently say that none of them were my long-lost twins. All of them had different life experiences and different concerns they brought to the work. Watch out for clients of similar groups to you who assume that you've had similar life experiences to them – "You're a woman/Chinese/gay/Jewish, you get it" – when you may not get it at all.

In summary: demographic factors may play a role in your connections with clients or they may not. The most relevant ones may not be the ones that you initially identify, and it's unlikely in any case that they'll tell the whole story.

Learning from outside textbooks

You will probably be required by your graduate program to take at least one class on multicultural competence (Constantine et al., 2006). These

---

1 Kleinplatz, P. J., & Ménard, A. D. (2020). *Magnificent Sex*. (Ed. Clare Ashworth.) New York: Taylor & Francis.

classes are a great opportunity to learn about big-picture concepts that organize our thinking about cultural differences and how they impact the provision of mental health services. However, great learning experiences about diverse groups can also take place outside the classroom, through less formal and, dare I say, more entertaining approaches. There's a lot of truth about the human condition in arts and culture, and I think psychotherapy as a profession ignores that to its detriment. Here are some thoughts on how to expand your understanding of the lived experiences of different groups and bonus, have fun while doing so:

- Consume art. Read books written by and about different groups, watch movies and television, listen to music, take in some plays or dances. Go back to your wheel of privilege and figure out which groups sit on the opposite side of the wheel from you, then pick a theme for the year with those differences in mind: "Fiction written by authors with disabilities" or "Movies with Black gay protagonists" or "TV shows featuring trans characters." Then read the reviews where other people from that group comment on the degree to which this art is true or useful; if there are inaccuracies in representation, and there often will be, consider what those mean for the group in question.
- Attend events. Put on your rainbow-themed clothes and go to Pride or attend a cultural festival specific to a country or group (e.g., Greek fest, Caribbean Carnival). These are great opportunities to learn more about groups directly and also to find out about and connect with organizations that serve these communities. And obviously a good chance to have a lot of fun, listen to good music, and eat excellent food.
- Stay current, using whatever means you prefer to consume news – websites, podcasts, radio. Printed newspapers are an option, I guess, if you're a dinosaur. Pay attention to what's reported, how the events are framed, and what's de-emphasized in the story. If there's a piece about challenges faced by members of a certain group, are their voices included in the narrative? You might also follow voices from different communities on social media to fill in the gaps not addressed by mainstream or legacy media. Spend a little time on your favourite social media platforms, connect with people from diverse groups, and pay attention to the concerns they articulate. Just limit the total amount of time you spend on these platforms lest you come down with a bad case of FOMO.
- Make friends outside of academia. Although I am hopeful that postsecondary settings are beginning to diversify the ranks of students admitted and professors hired, it's a slow process and a lot of departments are still demographically homogenous. You're far more likely to meet a greater breadth of people outside of school. Join community

groups that reflect your interests or hobbies like dancing, sports, crafts, games – whatever floats your boat (including, possibly, boats).

In curating your outside-the-textbook curriculum, think about which groups you belong to and which bubbles you may operate within from a learning perspective. If you are a gay Black woman and your social circles are predominantly gay, Black, or female, you may need a set of learning experiences related to non-gay, non-Black, and non-woman groups or some combination of that list. Identify your horizons and then try to expand on them.

If you're not angry, you're not paying attention

Nothing in my life has highlighted the challenges faced by minoritized groups more than working with people from those groups one-on-one in therapy. The stories I've heard are devastating, rife with all of society's worst "isms" and "phobias": racialized clients being bullied on the job, gay clients having homophobic slurs yelled at them from passing cars, and disabled clients struggling to navigate a world that can't be bothered to accommodate them. These stories are devastating to me, in two ways. They're devastating when the person is perfectly aware that the challenge they are facing is once again some racist, sexist, or homophobic bullshit, something they've likely been struggling with for most, if not all, of their lives. They're possibly even more devastating when the client blames themselves for a problem when I believe that it's not their individual issue at all but rather a systemic, social problem.

The main challenge, from my perspective, is that when you're providing psychotherapy, your role is to help the person in front of you, who may not be focused on fixing or overthrowing systems at all. I once worked with a young Latina woman, who was working three jobs to stay afloat and spending over two hours a day on the bus getting between them. I wanted desperately for her to find work that would pay well and let her use her considerable intelligence but for that, she needed a car, and she couldn't afford one on her minimum-wage jobs. My job was to help her process her feelings, find the joy in her life wherever she could, and find the energy to keep going so that she could ultimately break out of the intergenerational cycle of poverty that characterized her family history.

As a therapist, you must do what you can to support your clients who are facing systemic oppression; this might include changing their personal situation, fighting back against the system, or a mix of both, depending on the circumstances. Do what you can to connect clients to community organizations or resources that might provide tangible help with life problems like utility bills or finding employment. To manage your feelings outside of therapy, you can use your off-hours to support different groups through volunteering or making donations, contacting politicians or going to rallies or protests. Or maybe you will use your off hours to take care of yourself so that you can continue providing support to your clients. The key is to stay angry at the injustices you witness in session because anger towards the systems that maintain these injustices is meaningful and probably the only thing that will drive change in the long-term. Use that anger to explore how you do your job and the limits of what you can and can't do in a particular setting. Just make sure that you stay medium-angry: enough to fuel good work but not so much that you burn out.

On this issue, I try to remind myself of the words of Martin Luther King Jr: "the arc of the moral universe is long, but it bends towards justice" (King Jr., 1965). When I'm tempted to hand-wring about the state of the world or just give up, I need to be patient and hopeful and do what I can to support people in their own journey, trusting that the accumulation of incremental changes from thousands of people adopting the same stance will someday amount to real change.

Using microaffirmations to communicate allyship

In recent years, discussions related to diversity and discrimination have often focused on the impact of microaggressions, that is verbal or non-verbal interactions that convey discrimination against marginalized or minoritized populations (Sue et al., 2019). The flip side of microaggressions are microaffirmations: small acts that convey support and validation for members of marginalized or minoritized groups, affirming their dignity and humanity (Huber et al., 2023; Rowe, 2008). There's a growing body of literature focused on the role of microaffirmations in teaching and therapy; a lot of the research has focused on sexual orientation and gender identity (e.g., Anzani et al., 2019; DeLucia & Smith, 2021) but studies have also been done with members of different ethnic groups (e.g., Huber et al., 2021; Koch et al., 2022). Microaffirmations can also be intersectional (Boyce-Rosen & Mecadon-Mann, 2023).

There are many small ways to communicate microsupports and microaffirmations. Your options for decorating your physical space may be limited by your setting but if you can, consider adding pride flag stickers in visible places or putting your pronouns in your email signature. If you have a document directing new clients where to find your office in the building, make sure that your guidelines cover accessibility options. Ensure that there's enough space in your intake forms for people to write their full names and provide write-in options for questions about religion, gender identity, sexual orientation, and ethnicity. Use neutral language to avoid assumptions early on with clients like the word "partner" in asking about new clients' romantic relationships. And wherever you can, encourage colleagues to do the same.

Microaggressions towards the therapist

If you occupy one or more minoritized groups, or even appear to do so, I am sorry to say that you can expect to be on the receiving end of microaggressions from your clients. The research literature on microaggressions perpetrated against clients by therapists is growing by the day (e.g., Owen et al., 2014; Spengler et al., 2016), which is an encouraging development in the field. The literature on microaggressions perpetrated against therapists by their clients is moving more slowly but has received increasing attention in the last few years (e.g., Sackett et al., 2023).

As someone who has not been on the receiving end of microaggressions related to my demographics, my advice on how to manage this should be taken with a large grain of salt, if not an entire boulder. Know that your emotional response is valid and okay: if you are angry, sad, or scared, all of these reactions are fair and normal. You don't leave your basic humanity at the door when you walk into the therapy office and you're probably sick of hearing that particular flavour of nonsense from people everywhere, let alone from clients in your office. Take some time to attend to your emotions, whatever that looks like (see Chapter 5 on self-care). If you think it would be helpful, talk about the interaction with supportive colleagues or supervisors. Hopefully, you will have clinicians in your life who can speak to such experiences on a personal level but if they're not readily available in your immediate geographical vicinity, reach out to others through social media; the networks supporting clinicians minoritized on the basis of ethnicity, gender identity, sexual orientation, ability status, etc. are growing in strength and number every day. In all likelihood, you will need to address the comments or behaviour with the client as these are likely to interfere with the progress of therapy. This kind of conversation will likely be very difficult and you may be doubtful that it will do any good, which is fair. Change isn't guaranteed but it is possible. Depending on the nature of the client's micro (or even macro) aggressions, you may consider transferring their care to another clinician; if you foresee this possibility, it might be helpful to have a conversation with a supervisor or colleague early on in the work so that you're prepared if this becomes necessary.

Healthcare more generally and psychotherapy more specifically are fields that have long been characterized by cultures where providers are pressured to shrug off abusive comments from clients (Birks et al., 2018; Gillespie et al., 2010), but I think that is likely to change. The young clinicians I have been teaching and supervising over the past few years have very little patience for this garbage – quite rightly – and many call it out when and wherever they see it, whether from professors, peers, or clients. This seems like a long overdue change to me. We all deserve to feel safe at work, and that includes mental health professionals.

Subcultures

In addition to clients from mainstream cultural groups, you are also likely to meet clients who identify with certain subcultures: people who share common experiences and backgrounds, for whom that group membership has become a major part of their identity. The research on working with subcultures in psychotherapy is sparse but a few people have highlighted the challenges in working with different groups like police officers (Fair, 2009) or practitioners of sexual kinks (Sprott et al., 2023). Sometimes, subculture membership is based on a hobby or interest that plays an out-size role in clients' lives like alternative health practices or pickleball. I've found that clients in these groups are usually only too happy to share details about their activities, possibly in an effort to convert you, the uninitiated. You're unlikely to step on any landmines with these clients, but you will need to be careful that you are not dismissive of their interest. I've made that mistake before and in turn, received an earful about the transformative impact of pickleball.

Sometimes subculture membership is based on difficult life experiences and that's where there is a danger of stepping on clinical landmines if you're not familiar with some of the difficulties and challenges commonly experienced by members of that subculture. I'll use myself as an example here. My husband and I struggled with infertility and pregnancy loss for many years; the process of bringing our daughter into the world ultimately involved multiple surgeries, thousands of dollars' worth of medication, and a small team of medical professionals. Thankfully, there are many science-based infertility and pregnancy loss communities online who were enormously helpful to me in providing information, resources, and support during that time. Unfortunately, during my years of participation in these groups, I learned that even educated, well-meaning therapists are not immune to making insensitive remarks based on stories shared by other group members: "Just relax and it'll happen when you stop worrying!" or "You could just adopt" were some of the least helpful comments shared by others. The mockery of these therapists was extensive and ruthless, and I did spare a moment of pity for them, even as I felt sympathetic irritation on behalf of my fellow group members.

Unless you yourself are a member of a subculture or you spend a considerable amount of time immersing yourself on the experiences of that group, it's quite possible that you will stick your foot in your mouth when working with a client of this type. Much like dominant cultural groups, there's no way to learn the ins and outs of every subculture you may encounter and, in most cases, there's no research or best practices to consult anyway. Do what you do with other groups: learn what you can, ask questions judiciously, read up, be open-minded, and try to understand what group membership means to this person and what role that identity plays in their life. Just don't sign up to join the pickleballers, those people are intense.

Making a mistake doesn't mean you're a bad person

Making a mistake in any aspect of clinical practice is bound to feel difficult or unpleasant for the practitioner. "I have two brothers, not a sister," is always an embarrassing moment for a clinician trying to keep a full case-load of clients straight in their head. However, making a mistake when it comes to issues of cultural competency and identity can feel worse than other types of mistakes. One reason mistakes of this type may be difficult is because you know the client is sick and tired of being on the receiving end of these kinds of errors, as it is likely they've been hearing them for a life-time. You might also feel lousy because it might seem as though a mistake of this type automatically implies that you are sexist, racist, homophobic, transphobic, ableist, fatphobic, or some other brand of narrow-minded jerk. The thinking may go "Only a sexist person would use sexist language so if you've just told me I've used a sexist term, I myself must be a sexist and that would be just terrible." This is apt to trigger defensive and unhelpful responses.

We've all been raised in a certain place at a certain time within a certain set of groups, leaving us with beliefs, assumptions, and terminology about other groups that might be inaccurate, outdated, or just plain wrong. Most of us in North America at the turn of the 21st century have also been raised in oppressive systems and remain embedded in them, so sooner or later, you're going to make an assumption, use incorrect language, or otherwise miss the mark with a client from a group different to yours. Hopefully in this moment they *will* call you on it because that gives you a valuable learning opportunity, a chance to repair the alliance with that person, and the possibility to do better going forward. It's okay if your first internal response is defensiveness, just try to keep it in your head and not say some version of "Here's why what I said was fine and you shouldn't be upset" out loud. Take a literal or figurative breath before you respond. Apologize, listen to the client, read up on the issue after your session, and talk it out with other practitioners you trust to clarify your thinking. Have faith that these mistakes are repairable (Spengler et al., 2016).

Recently, I attended a workshop on microaggressions by a psychologist who is an expert in this area. She talked about the existence of "blindspots" for all of us in our language but lamented the use of the term "blindspot" as being potentially ableist. I have a suggestion for a replacement term: potholes. As in "I have some potholes in my use of language but I'm working on them." Potholes don't mean that a road is unusable or bad, just that it needs regular maintenance and upkeep. The process of discovering our potholes is often unpleasant but they develop inevitably over the long-term so the best thing we can do is try to fix them when we find them.

Trends in cultural competence

Keep in mind throughout your career that values, beliefs, and practices related to diversity and counselling are just as likely to receive regular updates as the rest of the field of mental health. In other words, you'll never reach peak cultural competence and not require any further education in the area. When I took multicultural psychology in graduate school, our professor helpfully informed us that "colour-blind approaches" – the idea that we would treat every client the same regardless of their race or ethnicity – were no longer supported, although it was unclear to me at the time whether they were ever supported by the individuals on the receiving end of these approaches. Instead, we were told, the new thinking was to develop cultural competency with a broad array of groups related to ethnicity, religion, sexual orientation, gender, and age. It was 2009, so there were a few major omissions to the list including non-cis gender identities, neurodivergency, and any mention of the word "intersection" to acknowledge the impacts of overlapping group identities. The relative impossibility of becoming familiar with the specific clinical needs of hundreds of different groups of people was not raised or addressed in the class. In any case, the research in psychology and mental health has largely focused on White, Educated, Industrialized, Rich, and Democratic (or WEIRD) participants (Henrich et al., 2010), so information about your group of interest might be lacking. For example, a few years ago, I was asked on short notice to meet with a client from Bhutan; as you might expect, the research literature is very short on studies about Bhutanese immigrants to North America and how they might present in therapy. Lucky for me, the client's main issue was frustration with their spouse, which is, I suspect, a universal issue to anyone past the honeymoon phase (see Chapter 8, couple therapy). More recently, the emphasis in mental health has turned to cultural humility, a stance of self-reflection related to one's own cultural biases and an openness to the client's background and experiences (Mosher et al., 2017). Cultural humility seems a lot more attainable to me than familiarity with every group you might encounter; more importantly, it feels more respectful of clients' experiences.

I'm sure you've snickered at some of the stories in this chapter (or possibly even guffawed) but know that at some point, your views related to multicultural practice will seem outdated too because that's just how the world works. Beliefs and evidence evolve and someday you'll be an old fogey wondering why the kids worry so much about an issue that was never addressed in your training. I think Patton Oswalt (2022) put it best:

> I'm woke, I think. But you know what? I won't be someday. And so will all of you. Be woke, be open-minded, just don't pat yourself on the back, because it will bite you in the ass…. I'll be doing comedy when I'm 70, and I will let slip something that I won't be able to keep up with. I'll be like, 'I don't think people should f**k their clones.' 'Boo!' ….No wait, I'm—I'm pro-trans.' 'F**k you, clone hater!'

While I think the piece about having sex with your own clone may not be relevant to psychotherapy, the rest of it feels very applicable.

Conclusion

When it comes to becoming more culturally competent, it may sometimes feel like you could spend your whole career learning and still not "achieve" competence. It's okay to have those concerns – this is never fully achieved by anyone. Working with clients from groups you might not otherwise come into contact in your day-to-day life can change you for the better, both personally and professionally. It's one of the real benefits of the job.

Chapter 11

Supervisor

A lot of mental health professionals spend at least part of their working hours at some point supervising the clinical work of students or recent graduates seeking licensure (Barnett, 2017) but most psychotherapy programs do not train their graduates in this crucial activity (Watkins Jr., 2012). The result is that many therapists arrive at this moment in their careers with a collection of traumatic memories related to their own supervision but little else in the way of preparation; in a desperate attempt to avoid making the mistakes their own supervisors made, they then go on to make a whole new set of mistakes. I know this because I have been a mistake-maker myself. Clinical supervision is a fascinating opportunity both to feel like a god of therapy gently initiating a group of anxious neophytes into the ancient mysteries of psychotherapy and also to face-plant in new and unforeseen ways in your attempt to train them. Let's discuss!

Preparing to supervise

Hopefully, your training program will have an entire course available on supervision as well as opportunities to engage in peer supervision and receive "supervision of supervision" (supervision-ception, if you will). If these opportunities come your way, take them, even if you think the provision of clinical supervision is a long way off in your career. At the very least, this training may help you better understand the process of your current supervisory relationships; at best, you can store up these clinical nuts for the future like some kind of clinician-squirrel. If you've already graduated or these opportunities were not available in your training program, don't panic. Caring about being a good supervisor and wanting to improve your knowledge and skills in this area is, if not half the battle, at least a very good start. Throughout my training, I had many wise, supportive supervisors who figured out how to embody the role through a combination of self-directed learning and experience rather than formal training; you probably have too.

DOI: 10.4324/9781003355366-14

After a few experiences of being supervised, make some time to sit down and think critically about what has worked for you, what hasn't, and why. Consider having the discussion with some classmates and possibly also some of your favourite libations and/or comfort food (you may need it). Use this thinking to identify your values for training others in the profession. Consider creating a supervision genogram (Aten et al., 2008), a symbolic representation of the experiences and relationships you've had with supervisors that gives you a visual map of the training you've had.

You may feel daunted and overwhelmed at the very idea of providing guidance to someone else regarding an activity that you've only just recently got the hang of yourself; however, I've generally found providing supervision to be less challenging than working directly with clients myself. It's much easier to make connections, notice patterns, and identify fruitful areas for intervention when you're not bogged down by the minutiae of a session. Plus you get to make ridiculous jokes and students are obligated to give you pity laughs, which is always fun.

Share your humanity

When I was a student, I marvelled at the ease with which my clinical supervisors made suggestions or interpreted the statements and behaviours of my clients. Godlike, they seemed, in their demeanour and probably infallible. On the one hand, this was reassuring – they knew the answers that I didn't and their sure hands were guiding the tiller of my therapy ship. On the other hand, it was wildly intimidating to try to share my mistakes and uncertainties in our meetings; as a result, I sometimes tried to avoid or downplay my own contributions to therapy missteps. I have a very vivid memory of the first time a supervisor shared a clinical mistake with me. As a student herself, a client shared an embarrassing sexual symptom in their first meeting, and she was so shocked and surprised by the confession that she laughed at him; unsurprisingly, this response was not well-received by the client, who was already embarrassed to be sharing anything about his penis with a pretty young female clinician, and my supervisor had to do some hard work to repair the alliance. As difficult as it must have been to repeat this story, her decision to share was enormously liberating for us students. If someone we respected as much as we did this supervisor could make such a mistake *and* recover, this might be possible for us too. What a relief! It became much easier in that supervision to share the messy reality of what was happening in session without worries about shame and judgement.

We've all made mistakes in our clinical work. All of us. We made certain types of mistakes when we started out, we made different kinds of mistakes mid-career, and we will likely still be making mistakes right up until the day we retire. Self-disclosure in supervision normalizes the process (Watkins Jr., 2017) and shows our students that we are not infallible gods of therapy (even if we wish we were). Likewise, share your self-care and your attempts to achieve work–life balance: if you're taking a day off or going on vacation, inform your students and discuss how you're planning to manage the boundaries with work, and don't then turn around and respond to emails like a big hypocrite! If you have a hobby or activity that you're comfortable sharing, bring it up and help normalize that our lives don't revolve around clinical work. If you have tricks for managing your to-do list, those are totally appropriate for discussion in supervision if you think they might be relevant and useful to your protégés. I believe that we can reveal ourselves as humans with our students, without being unprofessional, to everyone's benefit.

Preparing for the unknown unknowns – you can't

Supervisees don't know what they don't know, and there's absolutely no way that you as the supervisor can anticipate all the possibilities (Yourman, 2003). You can tell your students "Don't stick cutlery in an electrical outlet," and right away, they'll turn around and stick a fork in the outlet. When you ask what on earth could have prompted such behaviour, they'll say, "I didn't know a fork was cutlery." In training clinicians, there will be moments where it simply never occurred to you that anyone would do what they just did, so you didn't teach it or address it pre-emptively.

On one occasion in supervision, a student I had been working with in a hospital setting had had a less-than-productive meeting with their patient. When I asked why the student had not been able to connect as well as they had in previous meetings, the student explained that having the patient's family by the bedside during the meeting probably put a damper on the patient's self-disclosure. I asked the student why he didn't request the family go elsewhere and wait while he met with the patient. His response: "I can do that??" He'd been working at this placement for almost a year at that point and did not realize that politely asking family to leave was a possibility; moreover, I didn't realize that he didn't know that. I couldn't help but wonder how many of his therapeutic interactions to that point had been compromised by the presence of family members but alas, we could not turn back time (as Cher could have told us).

In these types of situations, don't beat yourself up when something goes wrong and definitely don't beat up on the student. The unknown unknowns will always be an issue in supervision no matter how carefully you orient new students or how extensive you make the documentation about clinical work in your setting. In recent years, I have told students that if I need to make a new rule based on an error they've made, I will be naming the rule after them, but I think that just stokes their creativity.

The main exception to the rule about letting go of the unknown unknowns is matters related to ethical conduct in clinical relationships. Do make sure that students have a solid grasp on the "tricky grey areas with no right answers" versus the "Please no, don't ever do that, not even one time." A colleague disclosed a traumatic supervision experience with me in which her supervisee shared some valuable information that their client had imparted earlier that day. My colleague said to the supervisee, "I thought you weren't meeting today," to which the supervisee replied that they had learned this relevant clinical data while taking a shower with the client that morning. This anecdote is undoubtedly the origin story of my compulsive need to remind my students on a monthly basis not to sleep with their clients, though I suspect I should probably broaden this prohibition to "any activities involving nudity and/or touching" to ensure that I have done my utmost to capture the fork/cutlery distinction in this situation.

Supervision will make you feel old

"I used to be 'with it.' But then they changed what 'it' was. Now what I'm with isn't 'it' and what's 'it' seems weird and scary to me. It'll happen to you!" If you (1) recognize this quote from Grandpa Abe Simpson and (2) are old enough to remember when *The Simpsons* was still fresh and funny, hope is already lost – I'm afraid you're over the hill.

This quotation to me represents clinical supervision in a nutshell. Therapy techniques and beliefs that were starting to fall out of favour and be seen as old-fashioned when I was in graduate school are now ancient history to my students: they've never even heard about no-suicide contracts, thought stopping to address rumination, or "colour-blind" approaches to cultural diversity. Similarly, therapy approaches and techniques that were seen as cutting edge and trendy a couple of decades ago are now not only mainstream but an expected part of the curriculum (e.g., positive psychology, third wave approaches).

I think the best we can do as supervisors is to understand that the evolution of thinking from "trendy" to "mainstream" to "outdated" is all part of the natural life cycle of the clinical ecosystem (Rief et al., 2022; Soares et al., 2020). You don't need to learn all the new stuff, just the pieces that are relevant to you. You also don't need to let go of all the old stuff – some of it is classic and evergreen, like Rogers' take on client-centered therapy (1951, 1961). Know also that some new developments in the field are likely fads and won't stand the test of time ("sand tray therapy", I'm looking at you). Do your best to keep up with the most relevant and useful of the new approaches but cherish the wisdom you've gained over time.

Address problems early

Most of us get into the helping professions because we have the personalities of Golden Retrievers (we want everyone to like us!), rather than cats (who cares what anyone thinks of us!?). As a result, I think a lot of clinicians have difficulty addressing problems with supervisees (Duff & Shahin, 2010), which is ironic for a group of people believed to be experts in fostering the development of functional relationships. We tend to take one of two approaches: (1) dish out unnecessarily punitive, heavy-handed admonishments or (2) sweep problems under the rug, cross our fingers, and hope the next training site will address the issues. Neither of these approaches is likely to foster growth in trainees or the clients they serve. We may avoid addressing problems with supervisees because we worry about using a sledgehammer to kill a mosquito or because we carry our own unresolved baggage about supervisors who were too hard on us in training. However, we can do trainees an equal disservice when we hold back (Nelson et al., 2008; Nelson & Friedlander, 2001). Finding the balance is tricky but some general guidelines apply:

- Don't attribute to malice what can be satisfactorily explained by confusion. Supervisees are learning a lot of information and skills at once, and some instructions are bound to slip through the cracks. Assume that they're just unclear and you'll maintain a more constructive relationship in the long-term.
- Be proactive. It's no use to say, "We felt concerned when we first observed this behaviour three months ago, but we didn't say anything at the time." While I certainly encourage you to give trainees the benefit of the doubt, no one finds feedback of this type useful. Rather, the first time you notice a problem, identify the situation, and suggest what be done instead: "I notice you did (this problematic thing). You need to do (that ideal clinical behaviour) instead because of (this excellent reason)." Often enough, this level of correction is enough for a supervisee who is genuinely motivated to do better. If the problem is repeated on subsequent occasions, you can then reference the previous conversations and reflect the existence of a pattern.
- Be as concrete as you can in your expectations so that the trainee knows when they've successfully made a change. Don't tell trainees they need to be "warmer" in session, tell them you want to see more validating and empathic statements and work with them to identify examples of what they could say and when they could say it. Give them a number-based target, if at all possible. Don't say "I need you to be more proactive in your communication" when you could say "Please email me

to confirm whether or not you met with the client." Be as specific and clear as possible.

- As always, document, document, document. If a supervisory relationship does become so problematic that it requires escalation to directors and other powers-that-be, it's always helpful to demonstrate the evolution of the situation over time and the attempts on both sides that were made to remedy the problem, for your sake and the supervisee's. If you provide corrective feedback orally, make a note of it in a supervision document. If you send an email to the trainee, save it. Hopefully, you'll never find yourself compiling a dossier of this type but if that stressful day comes, it'll be much easier if you know where your notes are (clinical life is always less stressful when you know where your notes are).

Use your clinical skills

The first time I taught an undergraduate class, I had some difficulty with a student who had elected not to follow the guidelines for an assignment and had done quite poorly as a result (note: if you are asked to provide five academic sources to support your arguments, *Cosmopolitan* magazine is not generally considered "academic".) Rather than see this as a learning experience and come to my office hours to discuss the confusion, this student had elected instead to take their issue with me to my head of department. I was complaining to my private practice boss, herself a former academic, about how ridiculous I thought this student was being and how stressful I was finding this situation. My boss listened patiently to this tale of woe and then gently reminded me that I was a clinical psychologist, suggesting that I apply my clinical knowledge and skills with this student. What personality traits was this student demonstrating? What coping mechanisms were they using? How was stress affecting their response to the situation? She encouraged me to think about how I would manage a similar response from a client sitting across the room from me and then apply those same strategies to the student sending me increasingly agitated emails. While my frustration didn't go away entirely, this advice certainly helped me to put the student's behaviour in perspective and respond more constructively.

Student trainees, like clients, can behave in a defensive, anxious, stubborn, avoidant, or over-confident manner (not usually all at once); they are therefore amenable to the same strategies you'd use with clients (Nelson et al., 2008; Watkins Jr. et al., 2015). Try using empathy, normalization, validation, encouragement, firm boundaries, and gentle challenges (probably all at once). I'm not suggesting that you cross an ethical boundary by appointing yourself as your supervisee's therapist but being humans, student trainees are likely to embody many of the same challenges. Feel free to use those hard-earned skills with both groups.

Clinical horror stories

I recently read *Hunt, Gather, Parent: What Ancient Cultures can Teach us about the Lost Art of Raising Happy, Helpful Little Humans* (Doucleff, 2021) because there's nothing us elder millennials like better than throwing out thousands of years of progress in favour of pretending we're cavepeople. Anyway, one of the strategies that the author describes is inventing monsters to help encourage good behaviour in children. For example, the monster who lives under the bed and gets bigger every time children leave wet towels on the floor, the demon who snatches up little children that don't get out of bed after they've been told three times, or the gremlin that bites the fingers of toddlers who won't leave their mittens on. The principle behind this strategy is that children know these monsters aren't real, but they're only 98% sure, so they're not going to take a risk on that 2%. The monsters are funny but also a little bit scary – it's a winning combination for enhancing motivation (in theory).

When I was preparing for licensure, I met monthly with a supervisor who had been working in the field for eons, and one of his favoured peda-gogical strategies was to share with me horror stories about the things he had seen and heard over the years from psychologists and other healthcare professionals. He was a treasure trove of scary stories and the lessons an impressionable young psychologist should take away from other thera-pists' lapses in judgment. Consider, if you dare, the psychologist who got months behind on their paperwork, was hit by a garbage truck, and was then subsequently fired when their replacement uncovered how behind they were in their notes and reports. The lesson here being "Stay up-to-date on your paperwork." Tremble when I tell you about the psycho-therapist who conspired with their chiropractor partner to submit false claims to insurance to fund regular massages from them, and who then got thrown under the bus when the relationship ended and the ex-partner got vindictive: "Don't try to scam insurance companies." Cower at the story of the psychologist who found herself on the receiving end of a complaint to her regulatory body because the man she was seeing was married and his wife decided to get creative in her revenge. I think the lesson from that one was "A lot of complaints to regulatory boards are later found to be baseless" but I'm not totally sure (maybe it was just good gossip). Were these tales true? Probably at least 80%. Did they include minor distortions designed to reinforce lessons into my suggestible little brain? I'll never know. But did they work? Undoubtedly – I've never committed insurance fraud, gotten significantly behind on my notes, or slept with a man who wasn't married to me.

Now that I'm a supervisor myself, I regularly deploy similar tales of horror to encourage good behaviour in my trainees. Do the students think I'm exaggerating? Maybe. Does it matter? Not if they get their paperwork done in a timely fashion.

"I thought about that thing you said" (supervisee version)

Students, like clients, are very prone to picking up on casual remarks. They'll ignore lovingly crafted lectures, carefully thought-out case examples, and beautifully explained interpretations and instead focus on that weird analogy you used one time when you were talking about case conceptualizations, where you compared clients' presenting problems to an octopus and asked them to consider whether multiple different issues were actually multiple octopuses or whether they were different legs on the same octopus.

For the concerned clinical supervisor, there are really only two options:

(1) In every interaction with every student, choose your words with the precision of a surgeon at all moments.
(2) Lean into the idea that as mental health professionals, we don't always know what will be most useful or will resonate best with trainees under our supervision, and that there can be great value in authenticity.

For people who have completed as much schooling as the average practicing therapist, it's an uncomfortable idea to sit with that we can't control how our words are interpreted and that our off-the-cuff BS may carry as much weight as our evidence-based pronouncements (Bachelor, 2013; Chui et al., 2020). The answer here, as it is in many places, is to hold your expectations lightly and accept the situation, despite the discomfort. Consider even that you could learn something about the most important aspects of clinical training based on students' fixations. You might discover that the most helpful learning you share in supervision doesn't come straight out of a textbook but rather out of your lived experience as a clinician, or that weird analogies are more easily remembered than straightforward comparisons. There's no way to know what comments in supervision will be the most useful so let go of the idea that students are enthusiastic little sponges who will absorb all your best explanations perfectly and without distortion. They're not and they won't.

Just recently, a student sent me an email out of the blue with the title "What I learned this year in CBT" and my first reaction to this declaration was "Uh oh!" After eight months of 3-hour weekly classes, I hoped desperately in that moment that her key takeaways might include a deeper understanding of the basic principles of CBT but alas, it was the octopus analogy. I'm still going to call that a win for the student's case conceptualization skills, and also possibly for her own supervision endeavors down the road.

Try not to take supervisee behaviour personally

From time to time, your supervisees will ignore your wise counsel. You've asked a student to write shorter session notes but every piece of paperwork you review from them looks like the outline for a Tolstoy novel. You've suggested they work on open-ended questions but the next therapy tape you watch in supervision is a litany of yes/no probes. You've recommended that they follow up on a therapy-interfering behaviour but several sessions on, this crucial conversation is still on their "to-do list." You might feel frustrated and wonder why the student is so willfully ignoring your pearls of wisdom. You have the key to cracking this case wide open and solving the clients' issues once and for all, dammit, why are they not taking advantage of this?

The answer is that students are rich, complex individuals with an array of motivations, values, and conflicting goals; there may be lots of different reasons for them not following your (obviously) brilliant orders. Despite your careful explanations, they may not understand what it is you want and are struggling to identify and explain where they perceive the disconnect. They may disagree with you on what to do and how with a client but not know how to communicate that disagreement assertively, yet politely. Sometimes the behaviour is part of a larger issue in the student's life that they may or may not feel ready or able to share with you, like anxiety or ADHD. Whatever the case, you may feel the urge to nag or scold in these moments, which is a completely human response to feeling frustrated but, in all likelihood, counterproductive. When I find myself in a situation of this type, I try to preface my comments with "Help me understand" because I feel that this frames the situation as a disconnect between the expectations of two generally well-intentioned people rather than something more malicious on either side.

Keep in mind also that some problems are self-correcting and don't require your intervention as a supervisor. For example, I've often found that students doing role plays with their classmates tend to be overly generous with one another by brushing past poorly articulated questions or unclear psychoeducation. In these moments, you may want to intervene and push them to refine their questioning or drill them on the wording they plan to use to provide explanations to their clients. Resist that impulse. Firstly, because it's not preferable that trainees go into their sessions with memorized explanations that make them sound like high school students performing in a play. More importantly, there's much better experiential learning to be had if the student fumbles their wording a bit with a real client: they'll ask their poorly worded question or offer some tortuous explanation of a therapy concept, and then the client will stare at them blankly and say "What??" Nothing sharpens the mind like having to reword on the fly under pressure.

Don't forget once you're a "grown up" supervisor that learning how to conduct therapy is very hard, and a lot of the early fumbles from trainees are the direct result of this exceedingly steep learning curve. Fixing problems at this stage in training can be like pushing down carpet bubbles or playing whack-a-mole. Beginning trainees will get the limits of confidentiality right but forget to complete the pre-session questionnaire with the client. In their quest to make more of their questions open-ended, they'll miss opportunities to practice sitting in silence with the client. Think back to the challenges of your own early days and treat them as you would have had your supervisors treat you – the nice ones, that is.

Share your unofficial wisdom

The entire thesis of this book could probably be summarized as "share unofficial wisdom" but let me make it explicit: whatever weird little tips or tricks you pick up across your clinical career, whatever noteworthy examples or esoteric learning experiences you've had as a clinician, share them with your students, even if they make you look silly, or maybe especially if they make you look silly.

Recently, a student I was supervising was struggling with her first therapy case. Whereas other students were puzzling out how to politely interrupt their chatty and sometimes tangential clients, this student had a client who defaulted to one and two-word answers; several sessions in, we had only the vaguest understanding of the client's problems and goals for therapy. In group supervision, we observed a tape from a recent session, and I watched as the student radiated energy throughout the clinical hour in her attempt to connect with the client but still made little headway. We switched off the recording and she looked at me with a pleading expression that seemed to say: "Tell me what to do with this client so I can make therapy work." I paused for a minute and said: "What you've got there is a cat client." "A cat client?" said the student. "Yeah, a cat client. Some clients are like dogs – they share everything, you don't have to dig to get the information you want, and the alliance comes very easily. You've got a cat client – you have to work harder, they don't just volunteer information, and it takes more time to build the alliance. You're not doing anything wrong, it's just their temperament and how they are in relationships. They probably do that with just about everyone in their life." Although I've never seen this type of client classification written up in an article or textbook, I have found it a helpful way over the years to frame clinical experiences; so did my students, judging by how often that analogy came up over the ensuing months. The client in question continued to be reserved and standoffish but the student therapist felt validated that this was not due to any failing on her part and seemed to be less self-conscious in session. The rest of the students had a great time attempting to produce other useful client classifications based on animals (birds, fish, and turtles were all identified as possibilities).

I am a believer in evidence-based clinical work, but I think the evidence base for clinical psychology is still pretty incomplete; there's an art and a science to this work, and it's sometimes easier to publish and teach the science than it is to communicate the art. Part of this art is the tips and tricks you pick up on the job so share those with your trainees. And look for our forthcoming paper, " 'Old MacDonald had a farm': An animal-based typology of client temperament and response to treatment" coming soon to a peer-reviewed journal near you.

You will let your students down

This is a uniquely painful lesson but supervisors are human too and therefore fallible. It could be because you're having an off day, because there's a personality mismatch with your trainee or because you've got a flaw in your supervisory game but eventually, you're going to let a trainee down (Nelson & Friedlander, 2001; Watkins Jr. et al., 2015). On that day, hopefully, they'll tell you and you'll have a chance to repair the rupture. However, I try always to remember that the power dynamic in these relationships is skewed firmly towards the supervisor, meaning that students won't necessarily feel comfortable sharing what's really on their minds with the person who can decide their grade, their success or failure in a practicum, or even their ongoing position in a training setting.

As I shared previously (Chapter 1, p. 10), the kinds of mistakes we make when we care about someone and want the best for them are different than the kinds of mistakes we make when we don't. Both types of mistakes hurt, obviously, but one type has more potential to cause grievous, possibly long-term damage. This is a very useful framework to keep in mind for clinical work, but it's also very applicable to supervision. If you care about supervision and you value the work, you will certainly still make mistakes, but they will be different than the kind of mistakes made by someone who is just checking a box and would rather be elsewhere. Intentions matter so forgive yourself when you misstep. If you do become aware of a rupture, you have a truly excellent opportunity to model making a repair of it, much as students might need to do with their clients or their own trainees down the road. Acknowledge the hurt, apologize genuinely, make amends, and explain what you're going to do differently going forward with that student in particular or with students in general. To extend the excellent advice that was given to me about clients in Chapter 3, don't yell at your trainees and don't sleep with them – everything else is fixable.

Teenager supervisees

In my supervision training, I was taught a model of supervisory needs and responses based on a developmental framework (Watkins Jr., 2012, 2017). In this philosophy, beginning clinicians need a lot of guidance, direction, and handholding. As time goes on and they are transitioning into independent practice, supervision becomes much less directive and much more on bigger-picture issues and overall professional development. However, right in the middle between those two stages comes the teenager phase. As a supervisor, I confess that I often find the teenager phase challenging.

Do you remember being a teenager? Did you feel like the adults in your life were hassling you all the time even though they were completely out of touch? "I know what I'm doing, mom!!" I'd say as I headed out the door to the mall, wearing my graphic tee and cargo pants, sporting a pair of freshly tweezed eyebrows, and clutching my flip phone. Looking back, I really didn't know what I was doing (especially in the eyebrow department).

Intermediate trainees go through this stage too. They know *some* clinical stuff. They've worked with a few cases, they've taken a bunch of classes and a couple of workshops, so they've got a handle on some aspects of practice. They're ready to test their wings and fly but you, goofy old supervisor that you are, you just won't let them. Ugh, what's wrong with you? Can't you just be cool?

This is a tricky balance. You do need to back off somewhat and give teenage supervisees the freedom they crave, but you also can't be completely taken in by their desire for independence or you'll miss some valuable training opportunities. I fell victim to this once with a student who had me convinced that she knew exactly what she was doing and didn't need my help; she would just report in, and I would passively receive the descriptions of her sessions. Half-way through what was rapidly becoming an unproductive therapy relationship I asked her, "Is this the first time you've worked with a client who has features of a personality disorder?"

She confirmed that it was. It would have been much more helpful had she shared this at the start, but really it was my job to double-check and find a way to address this in a way that wouldn't threaten her burgeoning independence.

Your teenage supervisees still need your guidance, even if they have a harder time sharing this with you than your beginner supervisees. Find a way to navigate their prickly exteriors and support them while you affirm that they definitely do know what they're doing in some areas. And maybe take away their tweezers.

Track your supervisory successes

I tell my students not to fixate on "a-ha!" moments in therapy: they look great in movies and television but are far less common in real life and not generally an indication that one session has been any more useful than another. In much the same vein, don't worry too much about "a-ha!" moments in supervision. More often than not, the clinical learning process is one of slowly building, understanding, refining, and adding to knowledge and skills than it is a sudden burst of insight.

Now and then, something you say will sink in and you'll see a new light come on in the eyes of your supervisees. They'll make a connection they hadn't made before or they'll truly understand some concept that's been eluding them. Try to catch those moments, if you can – point them out, both for your sake and your supervisee's. Similarly, a supervisee will sometimes reach out and tell you that you made a difference to them; on those occasions, save their feedback and document it for the bleaker days. Collate a file of thank-you notes or buy a fancy box to store them in if that fits your aesthetic (I'm more of a shoebox gal myself). These moments are so ephemeral and they're easy to forget so it's helpful to have an external reminder of why we do this work. And if this section moves you to send a thank you email to one of your past supervisors, I'm going to take partial credit for that little ripple effect.

Conclusion

Training the next generation of clinicians is an enormous privilege. What they learn about mental health and professional practice from you will carry forward. It's a chance to help shape their future careers, and by extension, their future clients' experiences. It's an opportunity to distill everything you've learned, sort out the terribly good from the just-plain-terrible and pass along some wisdom. If you do it right, you can reshape a student's entire outlook on the work. You're going to make a big difference to someone's career – never take that for granted.

Chapter 12

Virtual therapy

Like many other clinicians around the world, I was abruptly initiated into the mysteries of virtual therapy one very strange week in March 2020. When news of the pandemic went from vague reports to screaming all-capital letters headlines, I was working at a university student counselling centre. Our team had been told that we would likely be gone for only a few weeks, so I left my plants in the office and had to go retrieve them a month later when it was clear that our break would be much, much longer. A more prescient colleague brought her worm composting farm home that week in March, which is also how I found out that my colleague had a worm composting farm in her office for her lunch scraps.

At the time, I knew dimly that virtual therapy existed as a vehicle for delivering interventions and conducting assessments and that it might be a very good innovation for both clients and clinicians; however, like most other therapists prior to 2020, I had received no training in this interface. Not only did I have to learn how to do virtual therapy pretty much overnight, I started my current job as an assistant professor of clinical psychology just a few months later, so I found myself teaching a new generation of clinicians how to see clients using approaches I had only just figured out. In summary, the year 2020 was wild. I quickly picked up some of the basics but learned other lessons the hard way (for example, make sure your banana bread is out of the oven before you start a virtual session).

The upsides of virtual therapy (for the client)

Writing a section on why virtual therapy is cool in the ever-changing landscape of therapy-related technology feels like an anachronistic choice, like publishing a book in 2005 and explaining why this new fad for "texting" is kind of neat and might stick around. Future generations of therapists are probably going to read this chapter and say "Okay, grandma" while rolling their eyes and repositioning themselves more comfortably in the virtual armchairs on their holodecks.

DOI: 10.4324/9781003355366-15

Virtual therapy has a lot going for it from the client's perspective. For starters, it's convenient (Khan et al., 2022) – no driving or hopping on public transportation, no worries about finding parking or nasty weather, and no need to put on "leaving the house" clothing. Beyond these basics, for some clients, virtual therapy may be the only kind of therapy that works with their schedules: without needing to add extra time for travel and traffic, some people may be able to dig up 50 minutes somewhere in their workday or after work to see their therapist, which is especially crucial for clients with demanding jobs and/or time-consuming family obligations, i.e., the kind of people who could really do with the support from therapy. The value of this approach came into sharp focus when I did volunteer teletherapy for nurses and physicians in 2020: on several occasions, I saw harried healthcare professionals who used their smartphones to meet with me in their parked cars during lunchbreaks. Was this ideal therapy? No. Was it better than nothing? Definitely.

Virtual therapy also makes it easier for people who have chronic conditions characterized by pain, fatigue, or mobility impairments to attend (e.g., fibromyalgia, multiple sclerosis, long COVID). These clients may have enough strength to get through 50 minutes of talking about difficult issues with a therapist, but if they also need to add in all the extra energy required for preparing to leave the house and travel, they may come up short; see "*The Spoon Theory*" by Christine Miserandino (2003) for a vivid description of living with a chronic condition. If the cost of attending an in-person session is 9/10 on the energy scale, virtual therapy may be only a 6/10 and sometimes, that may be the difference between fitting it in versus not. Accessibility of psychotherapy is a crucial issue to address if we want to do more than pay lip service to equity, and virtual therapy affords us a valuable opportunity to practice this (Batastini et al., 2021).

Virtual therapy is also great for clients living in small communities who might otherwise be in a dual role with their provider. You won't have to have an uncomfortable conversation in session because the client teaches the only yoga class in town and doing adjustments in downward-facing dog has now become even more awkward than it was already (and it was always pretty awkward). It's excellent for mental health professionals who need therapy themselves but who would prefer to work with someone outside of their local pool of therapists, which might include past or future co-workers. (It's me, I did this.) Virtual therapy also makes it easier for clients to find someone who specializes in a particular problem or in a particular population; for some prospective clients, knowing that their provider is a specialist in a particular domain (e.g., supporting trans clients, working with polyamorous relationships) may be the crucial determinant of whether or not they seek professional help.

And then there's the actual clinical benefits. It's a truism in our field that clients will often cancel or fail to appear for their sessions on the days that they most need therapy, when the feelings that originally led them to seek therapy are at their most powerful (Barnes et al., 2013; Binnie & Boden, 2016). When people are feeling despondent or are paralyzed with anxiety, they often don't have the bandwidth to come to therapy to talk about it; this is a shame because talking about the pain in the moment that it is strongest may lead to much more powerful and useful sessions, and a correspondingly greater ability on the part of the client to implement changes (Tolin, 2016). Virtual therapy reduces the energy needed to see you, thus increasing the likelihood that you will be able to work on problems in the moment that the client most needs the help. Additionally, some clients may actually find it easier to open up and share during virtual therapy (Khan et al., 2022), which makes a lot of sense. Clients are likely to be more relaxed when they're wearing comfortable clothes, sitting in their own chairs with their own preferred beverages, and not feeling frazzled by traffic or worried about getting home in time to start supper. For others, the physical remoteness of the therapist may be a perk, rather than a liability: they may find it easier to open up to someone who is not actually physically present.

At the risk of making this book seem irredeemably dated, I think virtual therapy is really neat-o and anyone who says otherwise is a nincompoop.

The upsides of virtual therapy (for the clinician)

Virtual therapy has a lot of similar benefits for clinicians as it does for clients. Forget your dress pants, your pantyhose, and your pinchy work bras; with virtual therapy, you can wear elasticized-waist pants and adopt the "mullet" approach to workwear – formal on top, sweatpants below. If you're working from home, you probably control the thermostat, a wonderful benefit for someone who has worked in offices so cold that I occasionally had to run my hands under hot water to unfreeze them enough to write session notes. Working virtually often means that your kitchen and therefore your preferred snacks are more accessible (note: this is both a pro and a con). You also won't have to confront problems of traffic or parking or getting stuck behind garbage trucks, so you'll likely start your sessions in a much calmer headspace. If you're a very lucky person, sometimes a purring cat will set up shop on your lap and keep you company throughout your workday; more likely, they'll stare at you judgmentally from across the room, pausing only to lick themselves on camera at inopportune moments.

Then there's the health benefits for the therapist, beyond just decreased stress. Pre-pandemic, I occasionally had clients show up to their sessions with raging colds or infections, body fluids leaking everywhere. One time, I had a client come to therapy so delirious with fever from a case of the flu that I was unsure how many of me they were seeing. When I asked them why they hadn't cancelled, they looked at me, eyes crossing, swaying slightly, and explained that you don't ever cancel medical appointments for any reason. This was certainly valuable information from a clinical perspective and allowed me to produce a more thorough and accurate case conceptualization, but I didn't need to learn it so viscerally. I pity both the client and everyone they came into contact with on the bus that day. Similarly, the years I worked in hospital settings were marked by constant bouts of colds, norovirus, and strep throat, prompting my manager to say on one occasion to a bemused patient who overheard part of our conversation in the waiting room, "Dr. Ménard is cleared to work, but she's under strict orders not to lick anyone" (to be clear, I have never licked a client, strep or no strep). In the virtual therapy age, clients will usually email to say, "I'm feeling a bit off today, and I might be coming down with something. Can we take this online?" This is the perfect compromise between "well enough to attend and benefit from a therapy session" but "could still be contagious" and I, for one, appreciate the marked decrease I've experienced in viral infections.

Finally – and I cannot over-emphasize this point – virtual therapy often offers you the opportunity to see your clients' pets: cute dogs, adorable cats, maybe even a bird or two. Is this reason enough to switch entirely from in-person to virtual therapy? Yes, yes it is. In a decade of in-person sessions, no one has ever brought their cat to therapy, and my life has been less good because of it.

The downsides of virtual therapy

Let's take a brief detour from singing the praises of virtual therapy to consider some of the reasons that it has not become the default approach to therapy to date. Many of us pursue psychotherapy as a career because we enjoy the peace and space afforded by the traditional therapeutic hour, the opportunities it offers for genuine human contact. Our work is truly unusual in that regard: we sit quietly in the presence of another person and have a meaningful conversation with no distractions. Where else in our busy lives do we regularly make time and space for such powerful interpersonal connections? For me, going from in-person therapy to virtual was akin to moving from colour television to black-and-white, like watching *The Wizard of Oz* backwards. A lot of valuable verbal and non-verbal details were lost, and the quality of the connection felt poorer, a feeling that other therapists seem to share (Lin et al., 2021). There's something very distinct about being in the physical presence of another person that I don't think we've managed to capture by mutually staring at screens.

Part of the issue is that clients' non-verbals are harder to capture and read through the screen. A quick downward glance, a change in breathing, a tensing of the shoulders, a shift in position, a sudden catch in their voice – these behaviours and vocal inflections are harder to pick up through a webcam. The way that a person walks into your office, where they put their coat and bags, how they interact with objects can also reveal a lot of valuable clinical information. In one office, I kept a stuffed, sequin-covered snake draped across the back of my couch; when clients noticed, I told them that I practiced History-Informed Social Support therapy or "HISS" for short. Most clients ignored the snake but one young man who was using therapy to address his newly identified bisexuality picked up the snake and stroked it back and forth. Clients' interactions with objects are rarely so obviously Freudian, but they are often informative. Unfortunately, you lose a lot of this data in virtual therapy.

Another issue with online therapy is that powerful emotional reactions by clients in session can be difficult for therapists to address in the virtual space. In an actual office, when a client bursts into tears, I can hand the client a tissue box and lean forward in my chair while they cry. On rare occasions, I have touched someone's hand to help them ground them, helping them to refocus on the present moment so they can get some space from big emotions and reminding them that they are not alone with their pain. In virtual therapy sessions, I've mostly had to just stare quietly at the screen and do my best empathy stare, which is tricky to pull off. It may be important to remind ourselves in these moments of perceived helplessness that being present to witness expressions of pain and helping clients to navigate the aftermath of the emotional storm is more important than the form in which we are present, but I still worry that clients' experience processing pain in this way is less impactful in the virtual space.

I doubt that virtual therapy will ever overcome some of these issues completely. So far, I've never been able to recreate the same sense of intimacy and connection in teletherapy sessions, though I am hopeful that this may be possible as technology evolves. That being said, black-and-white movies, like the beginning of *The Wizard of Oz*, still have their place and their value.

Additional clinical details

I've had lots of clients misuse the term "hoarder" over the years to describe essentially anyone in their lives who falls closer to the "pack rat" end of the spectrum than the "Marie Kondo" end, so when a virtual therapy client described their parents as hoarders, I took it with a grain of salt.

Then they took their phone down to the basement of the family home and showed me the terrifying towers of stuff that threatened to tip over and bury the unwary visitor in an avalanche of junk. Yes, these people almost certainly met the criteria for having a hoarding disorder, and I saw the client's accounts of their childhood and relationships with their parents in a new light. Marie Kondo would probably have had an aneurysm contemplating that basement.

Occasionally, virtual therapy provides the opportunity to get more rich and vivid details of clients' problems than you might be able to get in person. The cluttered background of a client's bedroom might paint a more obvious picture of severe depressive symptoms than their verbal accounts. A client who makes the decision to attend a session in pajamas is providing the therapist with some valuable details about their capacity to understand and respect professional boundaries that might have been less apparent in person. In virtual sessions, you might witness clients' intrusive family members repeatedly attempting to barge into a closed room, and you'll also be in a better position to evaluate the exact words that the client has used to establish their boundaries with loved ones: "Please don't bother me until 2pm" versus "Why can't you assholes give me a few minutes of peace?!" I once had a client take refuge in their car to ensure the session was private and uninterrupted, only for family members to come and knock on the car windows. Virtual therapy represents a literal window into clients' lives and may provide you with previously unknown details relevant to their situation or illustrate the details you did know in unexpected ways.

Virtual therapy also invites us to *really* listen to what our clients are saying. Yes, talk therapy is theoretically all about talking and listening but virtual therapy can reduce the background noise and distractions so that we can more clearly hear the words clients choose, the pauses they leave, and the particular tone and emphases that they adopt in using those words. The absence of non-verbals is certainly a limitation to the work, but we can try to reframe it as an invitation to focus more deeply on the words themselves. Perhaps this is the main skill required to successfully practice virtual therapy: an interest in seeing what it can do for therapists and clients rather than a focus on what it can't do.

And returning to our consideration of how Marie Kondo's philosophy applies to psychotherapy, I don't care whether your paperwork "sparks joy" or not, you still need to do it.

Boundaries and virtual therapy

In many ways, it's easier to be professional and maintain appropriate boundaries when doing virtual therapy. There won't be any inappropriate touching between therapist and client because there won't be any touching at all. It's easier to start and end sessions on time when you don't need to collect and process payments and when your clients don't need to doff or don winter wear (a time-consuming behaviour in Canadian winters). Your client won't unexpectedly run into their sibling in the waiting room, leading to the exact conversation you might expect to overhear from siblings in such a scenario: "What are *you* doing here?" followed by "What do you *think* I'm doing here?"

In other ways, it can be harder to maintain boundaries in virtual therapy because you might be working in the place where you also eat, sleep, relax, do chores, and play. When we don't have to put on dress pants, pack a lunch, hop on a bus or get in the car to go to an office, it's easy for the boundaries between "work" and "not work" to get a little fuzzier. For example, after watching one session tape, I had to remind a supervisee not to wear workout clothes to do virtual therapy, even if they were planning to hit the gym afterwards. The signals of our surroundings can exert a powerful influence on our behaviour, and it can be hard to shift gears when your space is simultaneously cueing so many different roles of your life. Depending on the size of your space and how many people you share it with, you may not be able to set up your dream Instagram-inspired work-from-home space and defend it from roommates leaving their dirty dishes in view of the camera or children scattering toys everywhere. Taking a minute to check one's backdrop is probably a good start-of-day ritual for virtual therapy and might remind you to gather up those mugs with rude slogans and put them in the dishwasher (mine was a gift and says "I don't spew profanities, I enunciate them like a f**ing lady").

Appropriate boundaries can be a challenge for clients as well as clinicians. I used to joke when I started virtual therapy with new clients that we would all agree to wear pants[1] during our sessions. At the beginning of every session, I'd confirm, "Still in Ontario? Still wearing pants?" to check that they were in a geographical location covered by my license and professional liability insurance and that they remembered that this was still an appointment with a healthcare provider. Then a few months into therapy, a client forgot they were only wearing underwear under the blanket covering their lap and stood up to close a window. This is an important reminder on several issues: (1) habituation to messages received in therapy is an ongoing issue and should be carefully considered with respect to ethical principles and (2) a lot of people like to hang out pantsless in their own homes.

I hope that all of these issues will improve as the world continues to acclimatize to working online. After all, we collectively figured out how to

1 Trousers for my British readers, not underwear.

turn the ringers of our cellphones off during movies, so I'm confident we will eventually get a handle on this.

Noisy children and barking dogs – they're going to happen

The recycling truck in my neighbourhood goes by on Tuesdays. Sometimes in the morning, sometimes in the afternoon but always on Tuesdays. All of my students and colleagues are aware of my neighbourhood's recycling schedule because my dog has a blood vendetta against the guys who drive that truck. He's fine with the folks who drive and load the garbage truck as well as the people who drive the lawn waste truck, though I have no idea how or why he makes these distinctions, but the recycling truck guys are coming to kill us all and only his rabid barking will save the household from their menace. I've never had such a strong response in the chat window of the online undergraduate class I was teaching as the day I threatened to murder him on camera if he didn't shut up. Apparently, nothing I was teaching in an undergrad class about The Psychology of Sex was as interesting or compelling as threatened dog-icide.

Noise-related interruptions of this type are inevitable in virtual therapy. Be it pets, children, spouses, or neighbours who feel that chainsawing is the perfect activity to break up an otherwise dull Thursday morning, there will be uninvited noise at some point during your sessions. This is certainly frustrating and a particular downside to doing virtual therapy; however, as a field, we need to keep some perspective on the issue because in-person sessions are also prone to noise-related disruptions. In various student counselling offices, my September sessions were often disrupted by the loud music and screaming that characterizes typical start-of-the-semester activities. Construction, whether it's outside on the street or inside the hallways of your office building, is a year-round sport in Canada. Years ago at a private practice job, my office window looked out on the parking lot of a small shopping mall, where every Monday evening, all summer long, the local classic car afficionados would gather, play loud country music, and admire one another's cars – there may have been more to the ritual, but I was never invited.

There's not a lot of good, cheap options to deal with noise but do what you can in the way of installing soundproofing and acquiring white noise machines. Distracting dogs with treats at crucial moments is a possibility now and then but is not likely to be a viable long-term option for people who exclusively conduct sessions from home all day every day, as it is likely to result in canine obesity (although I believe dogs are generally enthusiastic about this technique). Children can sometimes be reasoned with depending on their age. I recall from my previous research (Kleinplatz

& Ménard, 2020) a participant telling us that Vaseline was essential to great sexual experiences: you put it on the doorknob to keep children out of the bedroom. This approach might not dampen the noise they generate on the other side of the door, but it would certainly discourage incursions into your therapy space.

I find that transparency is generally the best policy to implement with virtual therapy clients. If some noise might be heard in the background, warn the client and apologize pre-emptively: "My neighbour is chainsawing again, who knows why, but I'm sorry about it." I've found that most people understand because they've also got noises in their lives that they can't control. If you're comfortable with it, showing your noise-generating dog onscreen can go a long way to building clients' goodwill. And if you have a dog like mine with a personal beef against the recycling guys, maybe try to avoid scheduling your sessions for the exact hour the truck goes by.

Technical glitches – they're going to happen

I recently spent an entire lecture with graduate students in clinical psychology addressing the challenges of doing virtual therapy. I emphasized to the students that they needed to set up an alternate means of contacting clients in cases of technological failure. The last hour of our lecture was devoted to a guest appearance by a former colleague about doing assessments virtually in the context of private practice. Twenty minutes into a fascinating discussion, my power went out for the first time in years, and I had failed to set up an alternate means of contacting either the students or the presenter. The irony was palpable. Thankfully, this was just a short glitch and I was able to log back in, swearing up and down that this was a very purposeful illustration of the principles we had discussed earlier. Virtual eye-rolling from students is less obvious than the in-person version but just as devastating.

It doesn't matter if your office or your home has never, ever had a power or Wi-Fi outage over the last decade, you will have one as soon as you get involved in doing virtual therapy, so plan accordingly. Make sure that clients know your work phone number and you know theirs. Not to stereotype, but I expect some of my younger readers (cough, Gen Z, cough) may need to be reminded that their phone can be used to place calls. Put the plan in your intake paperwork and reiterate it to the client at the beginning of every session, if needed. Even if your own technology cooperates perfectly every session, the client's connection is equally likely to fail at some point. Have a back-up plan and make sure that your back-up plan is unlikely to also glitch out simultaneously. Therapy via carrier pigeon or smoke signals is tricky and you don't want to resort to that.

Mental health apps

Back when I was pursuing my year-long pre-doctoral internship, mental health apps were just beginning to take off as a concept; to put that time-frame into perspective, 2012 was the year the iPhone 5 and the Samsung Galaxy S III were released. I myself had a Microsoft Windows phone that served most of my smartphone-related needs, despite widespread and sometimes cruel mockery from friends and family for owning such a device, until it met a tragic end one night in 2017 when my dog chomped the hell out of it. Anyway, at the time, mental health apps were a new, exciting innovation and we were interested in how they could serve as an adjunct to traditional psychotherapy approaches. I had planned to do a seminar presentation about the offerings available for my fellow clinicians; however, between the time I conceived of this idea, and the moment several months later that we found time for such a meeting, so many apps had become available in the marketplace that it wasn't going to be feasible to cover even a small fraction of what was out there.

In the decade since then, mental health apps have multiplied across the various platforms like particularly horny rabbits. These days, there are literally hundreds of thousands of options available: trackers for thoughts, moods and symptoms, meditation timers, gratitude logs, little animated pets that die if you don't engage in self-care – you name the diagnosis, problem, or therapy intervention and there's likely an app for it. I'm particularly impressed by the apps that calculate how much the user spends on alcohol, cigarettes, or drugs in order to help them find the motivation to quit. I had one client who was able to stop smoking pot after many years of use when he realized he was smoking the equivalent of an all-inclusive Caribbean vacation every year.

The benefits of mental health apps to clients are enormous: even when their therapist is not available, they have help in their pockets whenever they need it. They don't need to carry around bulky photocopies of thought records or pull out coping cards from their wallets that are likely to become stained and damaged over time. Many of these apps even come with built-in alarms and reminders to track symptoms or complete activities, a wonderful innovation for clients who routinely forget to do their homework. The main challenge for clinicians in navigating this landscape is the sheer number of apps available, all of which vary enormously in quality. A client will roll into your office and tell you that they've been using the "Feel-better happy sunshine app" and you'll have no idea what they're talking about. Was it developed by clinicians and researchers? Is the content accurate and grounded in evidence? One recent review article of 5,000+ anxiety apps found that in over 2/3 of apps, mental health professionals hadn't been involved in their development and less than 5% had been rigorously tested (Sucala et al., 2017). This is not to say that such apps might not be of high quality and very useful to clients, but they don't have the built-in peer review system that exists for journal articles and books. There is just no way that your average clinician can stay on top of the giant pile of apps, and more are being created daily.

Your best bet if clients report they are regularly using a mental health app is to have them show it to you in session and explain how they use it. Hopefully, that will give you the opportunity to quickly review the interventions or recommendations built in and determine whether they fit with your overall treatment plan, or at the very least, don't undermine it. I have yet to encounter a "manage your anxiety by avoiding it" app but who knows what's out there? You might also get requests for apps that you personally recommend. If you use any yourself and like them, feel free to suggest those. Other good bets for finding quality apps are "best of" lists and recommendations produced by trusted entities like mental health organizations, university-based training programs, or professional associations.

I'm going to take a brief break now from book-writing to copyright the "Feel-better happy sunshine app" and hire some developers to make it happen. It'll be available for iPhone, Android, and Microsoft Windows phones.

Mental health and social media

This isn't strictly speaking about virtual therapy, but it falls under the whole "online, technology, computers" umbrella so I'm going to include it here. In his post-humously published book *The Salmon of Doubt*, Douglas Adams laid out his rules (2002, p. 95) governing our reactions to new technologies based on our age:

1. Anything that is in the world when you're born is normal and ordinary and is just a natural part of the way the world works.
2. Anything that's invented between when you're fifteen and thirty-five is new and exciting and revolutionary and you can probably get a career in it.
3. Anything invented after you're thirty-five is against the natural order of things.

This breakdown seems correct to me, especially as it concerns social media. I more-or-less understand the use and value of LinkedIn, Facebook, Twitter, and Instagram, all of which were founded when I was in my 20s. TikTok, launched in my early 30s, is a much stranger and more confusing place to me and I'm sure by the time this book is out, they'll be a shiny new platform that will seem pointless and bizarre to anyone old enough to remember Beanie Babies and "The Macarena."

In recent years, I've seen a lot more clients coming in with self-diagnoses based on information they've read online, most often from social media sources. Sometimes clients' self-diagnoses and the interventions they've implemented in response are fairly accurate and useful, or are at least perfectly harmless. At other times, clients may be partially or entirely incorrect in their choice of label or they may over-identify with a diagnosis to a level that's not useful. I suspect this is a new version of an old problem – mental health self-diagnoses come from TikTok these days but before that, it was Livejournal, and before that, it was lifestyle magazines. I suspect the Romans chiseled listicles of anxiety symptoms into the walls of their bathhouses when they found a few minutes between attending the chariot races and getting their new togas hemmed. Mental health and psychotherapy fads will ebb and flow even as the platforms where they are shared evolve over time. The main thing to do as a psychotherapist is to ask more about what the client has learned about mental health online and then gently correct misinformation as needed. And cherish your suspicions of technology developed after your 35th birthday: it's your right as someone rapidly approaching middle age.

Virtual therapy and AI

The text-based artificial intelligence system Chat GPT 4 was launched in the year I wrote this book, and there's been the usual spate of "this brand-new technological development will replace therapists!!" articles appearing across media sources. I'm not worried, for a couple of reasons:

(1) Breathless articles making wild claims about what brand-new innovations are likely to replace therapists are probably as old as the profession of therapy itself. So far, it's never come true.
(2) There was literally an episode of the television show *Black Mirror* about the feasibility of replacing a living, breathing human with an AI-enhanced bot. Spoiler: the real human ultimately rejected the inauthenticity of the bot's interactions with her and decided to store it in the attic, presumably with other miracle devices more commonly advertised on late-night television.

That being said, I do expect that AI is likely to play some role in enhancing the accuracy and utility of mental health apps or community support organization chatbots going forward. Just now, I told Chat GPT that I was feeling anxious about finishing this book and it recommended that I practice mindfulness and relaxation techniques, challenge negative thoughts, limit caffeine and stimulants, take care of myself through sleep and exercise, set realistic goals, and establish a writing routine, which is all quite accurate, if extremely generic, advice. It also reminded me to embrace imperfection, so any mistakes you may find in these pages were left in deliberately. I'm just doing what the AI told me to do!

Conclusion

It's a brave new world and some of it is deeply confusing to this elder millennial (too young to be a Riot Grrl, too old to be a Belieber). The increased awareness and understanding of virtual therapy foisted on us because of pandemic restrictions was a huge, if uncomfortable, step forward for mental health. I hope that many psychotherapy programs will retain and refine some of the online therapy training that was hastily developed in the face of COVID-19 so that new graduates may be proficient in both traditional and virtual therapies. I expect that virtual therapy will be a significant component of our future professional careers, which is going to open a lot of doors previously closed for both clients and clinicians. Some therapists might say that nothing will ever truly replace sitting down in a room with a client, face-to-face, and having a conversation. While part of me agrees with this, another part of me says that this format for doing psychotherapy is a luxury and a privilege that most people in the world can't afford or to which they don't have access. We need to meaningfully explore technology-enhanced alternatives, which includes virtual therapy, mental health apps, and possibly AI-enhanced chatbots. As I plan my clinical future, I fully expect that at least some portion of it will be online.

Conclusion

In 2020, I started work as an assistant professor of clinical psychology. A major part of this job involves training new clinicians, which represents both an exciting opportunity for me to shape the hearts and minds of the next generation and a fabulous chance to make a whole new set of mistakes and missteps. Look for volume 2, *Lessons from a Mid-Career Academic: How I Learned to Stop Worrying and Love Rejection*, on bookshelves in a few years. Part of the reason I made this career transition is that I have big dreams for how we should train aspiring psychotherapists. I think part of this dream would be fulfilled if there was a course in every single mental health training program called "Becoming a (good-enough) therapist." I've already mapped out the syllabus!

In this course, we'd talk about strategies that would help students sit in the therapist's chair more comfortably so that they could actually (gasp) enjoy their training. I'd remind students frequently that there are good reasons that they were admitted to this program and that they deserve to be here. I'd encourage students to set aside games of competitive one-upmanship and martyrdom in favour of supporting one another and engaging in self-care, both as individuals and a group. We'd talk about the impact of perfectionism on novice clinicians and consider practical strategies for how to address it. We'd normalize making mistakes in session and getting stuck with clients, as well as explore what progress and improvement really look like in psychotherapy. We'd explore fads and trends in the field of psychotherapy to decrease the likelihood of students shelling out $1,500 for airport hotel workshops. I'd help students to broaden their collective understanding on sources of "wisdom" as it relates to clinical work to include not only textbooks and therapy training tapes but also wise words from movies, books, songs, and animated Australian TV shows aimed at toddlers. We'd talk about the nature and purpose of clinical supervision and how to build safety, address issues, and repair disconnects in the relationship so that they could get the most

DOI: 10.4324/9781003355366-16

out of it. We'd discuss how to build networks with one another to support and enhance peer-to-peer clinical learning. We'd explore how impostor feelings manifest in clinical practice and how to manage those. I'd remind the students to regularly stop and reflect on the progress they've made in their clinical training and encourage their colleagues to do so as well, perhaps through a monthly discussion group. We'd identify the "start-up skills" required at the beginning of new placements and jobs and how best to develop them. I would encourage – no, mandate! – taking breaks of all kinds, including evenings, weekends, and vacations. We'd discuss whether continuing to answer emails while out of the office constitutes a break (I hope you know the answer by this point in the book). We'd map out self-care strategies and discuss how to set and stick to personal limits and boundaries and how to manage feelings of guilt that may come up. We'd explore the mushiness of the term "professionalism," acknowledge the possible validity of different approaches to embodying this across different settings and with different client groups, and consider the cultural embeddedness of the concept. We'd talk frequently about why none of us should ever engage in a sexual, romantic, or otherwise inappropriate relationship with a client and, importantly, how we should handle the situation if those feelings do come up. We'd definitely find some time for wildlife management strategies and other esoteric troubleshooting skills that might be required for helping professionals.

This class would also cover the transition into the world of becoming a "grown-up" professional, a.k.a. the adultiest adult in the room. We'd talk about building our clinical stamina and how to navigate the changes in knowledge, skills, and self-concept involved in making the transition to being a mental health professional. We'd identify and discuss the clinical skills and tweaks that are necessary for success in different settings, from private practice to forensic settings, addressing the challenges inherent to specific populations or workplaces. We would discuss expressions of stigma within the helping professions and how we might speak up when we hear others in the field using outdated terms or language. We would role play how to take payments from one another to better prepare for the world of private practice, though I don't think we'd discuss how to use the credit card imprinter. We'd learn about the scope of practice for different professions and how to cooperate, collaborate, and address disagreements on multidisciplinary teams. We'd talk about how to advocate for patients in settings where they may especially benefit from our voices. We'd explore how to cope when you lose patients, expectedly or otherwise. We'd consider how to creatively improvise with therapy techniques to fit the restrictions of different clinical settings. We'd weave EDIJ considerations and social justice efforts throughout the fabric of all our learning and discuss how we can work together to de-WEIRD therapy and mental health research. We'd discuss the challenges of supervision, and I'd encourage students to share their humanity with trainees as well as their unofficial wisdom and horror stories. I'd encourage more cheerleading across the entire spectrum: from supervisors to trainees, from therapists to clients, and from colleagues to one another. We'd talk about how to collectively participate in the brave new world that is virtual therapy and discuss how best to integrate mental health apps, social media, and AI in our practice.

Until such time as all programs put such a course into their curriculums, I would encourage everyone reading this to look for opportunities to implement some of these strategies in your own practice, in relationships with your colleagues, or as a clinical supervisor. My work now training aspiring therapists makes me feel hopeful and optimistic about the field. I see passion, deep caring, and energy in the eyes of my students to make needed changes to the field and to the discourse about mental health more broadly. I feel confident that the next generation will go on to shape a better world for clinicians and clients both.

Let me end this book with a very wise and deeply kind statement made to me by one of my first therapy clients, whose generosity in sharing this thought may have been responsible for me staying in this field even when I had significant doubts. "I encourage you to think about the good you are doing in the world by choosing to do this work." I would encourage all of you to do the same.

Appendix A

Recommended reading

Boynton, Petra, 2021. *Being Well in Academia: Ways to Feel Stronger, Safer and More Connected*. Routledge.

Cozolino, Louis, 2004. *The Making of a Therapist: A Practical Guide for the Inner Journey*. W.W. Norton & Company.

Dalgleish, Tracy, 2023. *I Didn't Sign Up for This*. Pesi Publishing.

Hoyt, Michael F. (ed.), 2013. *Therapist Stories of Inspiration, Passion & Renewal*. Routledge.

Kottler, Jeffrey, 2017. *On Being a Therapist*, 5th edition. Oxford University Press.

Pipher, Mary, 2016. *Letters to a Young Therapist*, Revised edition. Basic Books.

Yalom, Irvin D., reissued 2017. *The Gift of Therapy*. Harper Collins.

Aphorisms for the clinician in a hurry

- You are not a worse therapist than all your classmates.
- Always pee before your sessions.
- Keep a cardigan in your office.
- Document, document, document.
- Don't have sex with your clients.
- Transparency with clients will get you a long way.
- With trainees, don't attribute to malice what can be satisfactorily explained by inexperience.
- With clients, don't attribute to malice what can be satisfactorily explained by boredom.
- The time to do self-care is before you're in need of it.
- No seriously, do NOT have sex with your clients. Ever.
- One supervisor's "unprofessional outfit" is another supervisor's "cute look."
- For periods of intense life stress: when in doubt, dial back.
- For self-disclosure with clients: when in doubt, dial back.
- Respect your own work boundaries as you would have clients respect theirs.
- Don't have sex with your supervisees.
- You could be the right therapist at the right time.
- You could also be the right therapist at the wrong time.
- If you do teletherapy, you will have technical difficulties. Plan accordingly.
- For patients with tough or complex problems: don't assume you will make a difference and don't assume you won't.
- Your supervisees may sometimes remind you of teenagers – that's normal.
- Run the mile you're in.
- Ask yourself "What Would A Good-Enough Therapist Do?" (WWAGETD?)

References

Adames, H. Y., Chavez-Dueñas, N. Y., Vasquez, M. J. T., & Pope, K. S. (2022). Addressing the hazards of lonliness. In *Succeeding as a therapist: How to create a thriving practice in a changing worlds*. American Psychological Association.

Adams, D. (2002). *The salmon of doubt*. Pocket Books.

American Psychological Association. (2003). Guidelines on multicultural education, training, research, practice, and organizational change for psychologists. *American Psychologist*, 58(5), 377–402. https://doi.org/10.1037/0003-066X.58.5.377

Anzani, A., Morris, E. R., & Galupo, M. P. (2019). From absence of microaggressions to seeing authentic gender: Transgender clients' experiences with microaffirmations in therapy. *Journal of LGBT Issues in Counseling*, 13(4), 258–275. https://doi.org/10.1080/15538605.2019.1662359

Apostolou, M., Christoforou, C., & Lajunen, T. J. (2023). What are romantic relationships good for? An explorative analysis of the perceived benefits of being in a relationship. *Evolutionary Psychology*, 21(4), 1–11. https://doi.org/10.1177/14747049231210245

Ashcroft, R., Kourgiantakis, T., Fearing, G., Robertson, T., & Brown, J. B. (2019). Social work's scope of practice in primary mental health care: A scoping review. *British Journal of Social Work*, 49(2), 318–334. https://doi.org/10.1093/bjsw/bcy051

Aten, J. D., Madson, M. B., & Kruse, S. J. (2008). The supervision genogram: A tool for preparing supervisors-in-training. *Psychotherapy*, 45(1), 111–116.

Auden, W. H. (1962). *The Dyer's hand and other essays*. Random House.

Bachelor, A. (2013). Clients' and therapists' views of the therapeutic alliance: Similarities, differences and relationship to therapy outcome. *Clinical Psychology and Psychotherapy*, 20(2), 118–135. https://doi.org/10.1002/cpp.792

Baier, A. L., Kline, A. C., & Feeny, N. C. (2020). Therapeutic alliance as a mediator of change: A systematic review and evaluation of research. *Clinical Psychology Review*, 82, 1–14. https://doi.org/10.1016/j.cpr.2020.101921

Bailin, A., Bearman, S. K., & Sale, R. (2018). Clinical supervision of mental health professionals serving youth: Format and microskills. *Administration and Policy in Mental Health and Mental Health Services Research*, 45(5), 800–812. https://doi.org/10.1007/s10488-018-0865-y

Barnes, M., Sherlock, S., Thomas, L., Kessler, D., Kuyken, W., Owen-Smith, A., Lewis, G., Wiles, N., & Turner, K. (2013). No pain, no gain: Depressed clients' experiences of cognitive behavioural therapy. *British Journal of Clinical Psychology*, 52(4), 347–364. https://doi.org/10.1111/bjc.12021

Barnett, J. E. (2017). Becoming a clinical supervisor: Key ethics issues and recommendations. *Journal of Health Service Psychology*, 10–18.

Barnett, J. E., & Molzon, C. H. (2014). Clinical supervision of psychotherapy: Essential ethics issues for supervisors and supervisees. *Journal of Clinical Psychology*, 70(11), 1051–1061. https://doi.org/10.1002/jclp.22126

Basa, V. (2019). Peer supervision in the therapeutic field. *European Journal of Counselling Theory, Research and Practice*, 3, 1–10.

Batastini, A. B., Paprzycki, P., Jones, A. C. T., & MacLean, N. (2021). Are videoconferenced mental and behavioral health services just as good as in-person? A meta-analysis of a fast-growing practice. *Clinical Psychology Review*, 83, 1–22. https://doi.org/10.1016/j.cpr.2020.101944

Binnie, J., & Boden, Z. (2016). Non-attendance at psychological therapy appointments. *Mental Health Review Journal*, 21(3), 231–248. https://doi.org/10.1108/MHRJ-12-2015-0038

Birks, M., Budden, L. M., Biedermann, N., Park, T., & Chapman, Y. (2018). A 'rite of passage?': Bullying experiences of nursing students in Australia. *Collegian*, 25(1), 45–50. https://doi.org/10.1016/j.colegn.2017.03.005

Blanchard, M., & Farber, B. A. (2020). "It is never okay to talk about suicide": Patients' reasons for concealing suicidal ideation in psychotherapy. *Psychotherapy Research*, 30(1), 124–136. https://doi.org/10.1080/10503307.2018.1543977

Bohart, A. C., & Tallman, K. (2010). Clients: The neglected common factor in psychotherapy. In B. L. Duncan, S. C. Miller, B. E. Wampold, & M. A. Hubble (Eds.), *Heart and soul of change: Delivering what works in therapy* (pp. 83–112). American Psychological Association. https://doi.org/10.1037/12075-003

Bokhof, B., & Junius-Walker, U. (2016). Reducing polypharmacy from the perspectives of general practitioners and older patients: A synthesis of qualitative studies. *Drugs and Aging*, 33(4), 249–266. https://doi.org/10.1007/s40266-016-0354-5

Bonitz, V. (2008). Use of physical touch in the "talking cure": A journey to the outskirts of psychotherapy. *Psychotherapy Theory, Research, Practice, Training*, 45(3), 391–404. https://doi.org/10.1037/a0013311

Booth, A., Scantlebury, A., Hughes-Morley, A., Mitchell, N., Wright, K., Scott, W., & McDaid, C. (2017). Mental health training programmes for non-mental health trained professionals coming into contact with people with mental ill health: A systematic review of effectiveness. *BMC Psychiatry*, 17(1), 1–24. https://doi.org/10.1186/s12888-017-1356-5

Borders, L. D. A., Dianna, J. A., & McKibben, W. B. (2023). Clinical supervisor training: a ten-year scoping review across counseling, psychology, and social work. *Clinical Supervisor*, 42(1), 164–212. https://doi.org/10.1080/07325 223.2023.2188624

Bowie, C., McLeod, J., & McLeod, J. (2016). 'It was almost like the opposite of what I needed': A qualitative exploration of client experiences of unhelpful therapy. *Counselling and Psychotherapy Research*, 16(2), 79–87. https://doi.org/10.1002/capr.12066

Boyce-Rosen, N., & Mecadon-Mann, M. (2023). Microaffirmations: Small gestures toward equity and advocacy. *Professional School Counseling*, 27(1a), 1–10. https://doi.org/10.1177/2156759x231160722

Braithwaite, S., & Holt-Lunstad, J. (2017). Romantic relationships and mental health. In G. C. Karantzas, J. A. Simpson, & M. P. McCabe (Eds.), *Current Opinion in Psychology* (Vol. 13, pp. 120–125). Elsevier. https://doi.org/10.1016/j.copsyc.2016.04.001

Bray, B. (2019). Counselor self-disclosure: Encouragement or impediment to client growth? *Counseling Today*. Retrieved from www.counseling.org/publications/counseling-today-magazine/article-archive/article/legacy/counselor-self-disclosure-encouragement-or-impediment-to-client-growth

Britton, J., & Propper, C. (2016). Teacher pay and school productivity: Exploiting wage regulation. *Journal of Public Economics*, 133, 75–89. https://doi.org/10.1016/j.jpubeco.2015.12.004

Brown, J., Lewis, L., Ellis, K., Stewart, M., Freeman, T. R., & Kasperski, M. J. (2011). Conflict on interprofessional primary health care teams can it be resolved? *Journal of Interprofessional Care*, 25(1), 4–10. https://doi.org/10.3109/13561820.2010.497750

Byers, E. S., Henderson, J., & Hobson, K. M. (2009). University students' definitions of sexual abstinence and having sex. *Archives of Sexual Behavior*, 38(5), 665–674. https://doi.org/10.1007/s10508-007-9289-6

Cain, S. (2012). *Quiet: The power of introverts in a world that can't stop talking*. Crown.

Caldwell, B. (2018). Is it couple, couples, or couple's therapy? *Psychotherapy Notes*. Retrieved from www.psychotherapynotes.com/couple-therapy-couples-therapy/

Catterson, A., Gautam, M., Kerr, P. J., Pecher, M., Waiser, D., & Kaji, J. (1997). A cross-sectional study of private psychiatric practices sunder a single-payer health care system. *Canadian Journal of Psychiatry*, 42, 395–401.

Caulfield, T. (2015). *The science of celebrity…or is Gwyneth Paltrow wrong about everything?* Penguin Canada.

Caulfield, A., Vatansever, D., Lambert, G., & Van Bortel, T. (2019). WHO guidance on mental health training: A systematic review of the progress for non-specialist health workers. *BMJ Open*, 9(1), 1–16. https://doi.org/10.1136/bmjopen-2018-024059

Chait Barnett, R., Steptoe, A., & Gareis, K. C. (2005). Marital-role quality and stress-related psychobiological indicators. *Annals of Behavioral Medicine*, 30(1), 36–43.

Chang, D. F., & Berk, A. (2009). Making cross-racial therapy work: A phenomenological study of clients' experiences of cross-racial therapy. *Journal of Counseling Psychology*, 56(4), 521–536. https://doi.org/10.1037/a0016905

Chang, L.-Y., Yu, H.-H., & Chao, Y.-F. (2019). The relationship between nursing workload, quality of care, and nursing payment in intensive care units. *Journal of Nursing Research*, 21(1), 1–9.

Chemtob, C. M., Hamada, R. S., Bauer, G., Torigoe, R. Y., & Kinney, B. (1988). Patient suicide: Frequency and impact on psychologists. *Professional Psychology: Research and Practice*, 19(4), 416–420.

Chui, H., Palma, B., Jackson, J. L., & Hill, C. E. (2020). Therapist-client agreement on helpful and wished-for experiences in psychotherapy: Associations with outcome. *Journal of Counseling Psychology*, 67(3), 349–360. https://doi.org/10.1037/cou0000393

Clance, P. R. (1985).Clance Impostor Phenomenon Scale (CIPS) [Database record]. APA PsycTests. https://doi.org/10.1037/t11274-000

Clance, P. R., & Imes, S. (1978). The Imposter Phenomenon in high achieving women: Dynamics and therapeutic intervention. *Psychotherapy Theory, Research and Practice*, 15(3), 1–8.

College of Psychologists of Ontario. (2017). *Standards of Professional Conduct.*

Constantine, T. B., Dunn, M. G., Dinehart, T. M., & Montoya, J. A. (2006). Multicultural education in the mental health professions: A meta-analytic review. *Journal of Counseling Psychology*, 53, 132–145. https://scholarsarchive.byu.edu/facpubhttps://scholarsarchive.byu.edu/facpub/2028

Cooper, M. (2008). *Essential research findings in counselling & psychotherapy.* SAGE Publications.

Crits-Christoph, P., Gibbons, M. B. C., Barber, J. P., Gallop, R., Beck, A. T., Mercer, D., Tu, X., Weiss, R. D., Thase, M. E., & Frank, A. (2003). Mediators of outcome of psychosocial treatments for cocaine dependence. *Journal of Consulting and Clinical Psychology*, 71(5), 918–925. https://doi.org/10.1037/0022-006X.71.5.918

Dalgleish, T. (2023). *I didn't sign up for this: A couples therapist shares real-life stories of breaking patterns and finding joy in relationships…including her own.* PESI Publishing, Inc.

Damon, H., Ayling, R., & Lodge, R. (2022). A constructivist grounded theory of counselling psychologists' in-the-moment decision-making process about touching their clients. *Counselling Psychology Review*, 37(2), 37–46.

Darden, A. J., & Rutter, P. A. (2011). Psychologists' experiences of grief after client suicide: A qualitative study. *Omega: Journal of Death and Dying*, 63(4), 317–342. https://doi.org/10.2190/OM.63.4.b

DeLucia, R., & Smith, N. G. (2021). The impact of provider biphobia and microaffirmations on bisexual individuals' treatment-seeking intentions. *Journal of Bisexuality*, 21(2), 145–166. https://doi.org/10.1080/15299716.2021.1900020

Dembowsky, A. (2016). Psychotherapists gravitated toward patients who can pay. *PBS.* Retrieved from www.pbs.org/newshour/health/psychotherapists-gravitate-toward-patients-can-pay

Doherty, W. J., Harris, S. M., Hall, E. L., & Hubbard, A. K. (2021). How long do people wait before seeking couples therapy? A research note. *Journal of Marital and Family Therapy*, 47(4), 882–890. https://doi.org/10.1111/jmft.12479

Doss, B. D., Thum, Y. M., Sevier, M., Atkins, D. C., & Christensen, A. (2005). Improving relationships: Mechanisms of change in couple therapy. *Journal of Consulting and Clinical Psychology, 73*(4), 624–633. https://doi.org/10.1037/0022-006X.73.4.624

Doucleff, M. (2021). *Hunt, gather, parent: What ancient cultures can teach us about the lost art of raising happy, helpful little humans.* Simon & Schuster.

Drouin, M., Coupe, M., & Temple, J. R. (2017). Is sexting good for your relationship? It depends .... *Computers in Human Behavior, 75,* 749–756. https://doi.org/10.1016/j.chb.2017.06.018

Duckworth, S. (2020, Oct 18). Wheel of power/privilege [Infographic]. Flickr. Retrieved from www.flickr.com/photos/sylviaduckworth/50500299716/.

Duff, C. T., & Shahin, J. (2010). Conflict in clinical supervision: Antecedents, impact, amelioration, and prevention. *The Alberta Counselor, 31*(1), 3–8.

Duncan, R. E., Hall, A. C., & Knowles, A. (2015). Ethical dilemmas of confidentiality with adolescent clients: Case studies from psychologists. *Ethics and Behavior, 25*(3), 197–221. https://doi.org/10.1080/10508422.2014.923314

Elizabeth, J., & Callaghan, M. (2005). Becoming a psychologist: professionalism, feminism, activism. *Annual Review of Critical Psychology, 4,* 139–153. www.researchgate.net/publication/51014568

Eubanks, C. F., Sergi, J., Samstag, L. W., & Muran, J. C. (2021). Commentary: Rupture repair as a transtheoretical corrective experience. *Journal of Clinical Psychology, 77*(2), 457–466. https://doi.org/10.1002/jclp.23117

Fair, D. J. (2009). Counseling cops learning how to navigate the law. *Annals of the American Psychotherapy Association, 12*(4), 50–51.

Falconer, T., & Humphreys, T. P. (2019). Sexting outside the primary relationship: Prevalence, relationship influences, physical engagement, and perceptions of "cheating." *Canadian Journal of Human Sexuality, 28*(2), 134–142. https://doi.org/10.3138/cjhs.2019-0011

Falender, C. A., & Shafranske, E. P. (2012). The importance of competency-based clinical supervision and training in the twenty-first century: Why bother? *Journal of Contemporary Psychotherapy, 42*(3), 129–137. https://doi.org/10.1007/s10879-011-9198-9

Falender, C. A., & Shafranske, E. P. (2014). Clinical supervision: The state of the art. *Journal of Clinical Psychology, 70*(11), 1030–1041. https://doi.org/10.1002/jclp.22124

Falender, C. A., & Shafranske, E. P. (2017). Competency-based clinical supervision: Status, opportunities, tensions, and the future. *Australian Psychologist, 52*(2), 86–93. https://doi.org/10.1111/ap.12265

Finlayson, M., & Graetz Simmonds, J. (2018). Impact of client suicide on psychologists in Australia. *Australian Psychologist, 53*(1), 23–32. https://doi.org/10.1111/ap.12240

Fraenkel, P. (2019). Love in action: An integrative approach to last chance couple therapy. *Family Process, 58*(3), 569–594. https://doi.org/10.1111/famp.12474

Friedlander, M. L., Angus, L., Wright, S. T., Günther, C., Austin, C. L., Kangos, K., Barbaro, L., Macaulay, C., Carpenter, N., & Khattra, J. (2018). "If those tears could talk, what would they say?" Multi-method analysis of a corrective experience in brief dynamic therapy. *Psychotherapy Research*, *28*(2), 217–234. https://doi.org/10.1080/10503307.2016.1184350

Gillespie, G. L., Gates, D. M., Miller, M., & Kunz Howard, P. (2010). Violence against healthcare workers in a pediatric emergency department. *Advanced Emergency Nursing Journal*, *32*(1), 68–82.

Global Wellness Institute (2023). *The Global Wellness Economy Monitor 2023*. Retrieved from https://globalwellnessinstitute.org/the-2023-global-wellness-economy-monitor/

Golia, G. M., & McGovern, A. R. (2015). If you save me, i'll save you: The power of peer supervision in clinical training and professional development. *British Journal of Social Work*, *45*(2), 634–650. https://doi.org/10.1093/bjsw/bct138

Goodyear, R., Lichtenberg, J., Hutman, H., Overland, E., Bedi, R., Christiani, K., Di Mattia, M., du Preez, E., Farrell, B., Feather, J., Grant, J., Han, Y., Ju, Y., Lee, D., Lee, H., Nicholas, H., Jones Nielsen, J., Sinacore, A., Tu, S., & Young, C. (2016). A global portrait of counselling psychologists' characteristics, perspectives, and professional behaviors. *Counselling Psychology Quarterly*, *29*(2), 115–138. https://doi.org/10.1080/09515070.2015.1128396

Gottlieb, M. C., Lasser, J., & Simpson, G. L. (2008). Legal and ethical issues in couple therapy. In A. S. Gurman (Ed.), *Clinical handbook of couple therapy* (4th ed., pp. 698–717). Guildford Press.

Gray, D. P., Dineen, M., & Sidaway-Lee, K. (2020). The worried well. *British Journal of General Practice*, *70*(691), 84–85. https://doi.org/10.3399/bjgp20 X708017

Greenberg, R. P., Constantino, M. J., & Bruce, N. (2006). Are patient expectations still relevant for psychotherapy process and outcome? *Clinical Psychology Review*, *26*(6), 657–678. https://doi.org/10.1016/j.cpr.2005.03.002

Hall, W. J., Chapman, M. V., Lee, K. M., Merino, Y. M., Thomas, T. W., Payne, B. K., Eng, E., Day, S. H., & Coyne-Beasley, T. (2015). Implicit racial/ethnic bias among health care professionals and its influence on health care outcomes: A systematic review. *American Journal of Public Health*, *105*(12), 60–76. https://doi.org/10.2105/AJPH.2015.302903

Hanson, J. (2005). Should your lips be zipped? How therapist self-disclosure and non-disclosure affects clients. *Counselling and Psychotherapy Research*, *5*(2), 96–104. https://doi.org/10.1080/17441690500226658

Hayes, S.C., Strosahl, K., & Wilson, K.G. (1999). *Acceptance and Commitment Therapy: An experiential approach to behavior change*. Guilford Press.

Heinonen, E., & Orlinsky, D. E. (2013). Psychotherapists' personal identities, theoretical orientations, and professional relationships: Elective affinity and role adjustment as modes of congruence. *Psychotherapy Research*, *23*(6), 718–731. https://doi.org/10.1080/10503307.2013.814926

Henrich, J., Heine, S. J., & Norenzayan, A. (2010). The weirdest people in the world? *Behavioral and Brain Sciences*, *33*(2–3), 61–83. https://doi.org/10.1017/S0140525X0999152X

Hill, C. E., Lystrup, A., Kline, K., Gebru, N. M., Birchler, J., Palmer, G., Robinson, J., Um, M., Griffin, S., Lipsky, E., Knox, S., & Pinto-Coelho, K. (2013). Aspiring to become a therapist: Personal strengths and challenges, influences, motivations, and expectations of future psychotherapists. *Counselling Psychology Quarterly*, 26(3–4), 267–293. https://doi.org/10.1080/09515070.2013.825763

Hodges, B., Paul, R., & Ginsburg, S. (2019). Assessment of professionalism: From where have we come–to where are we going? An update from the Ottawa Consensus Group on the assessment of professionalism. *Medical Teacher*, 41(3), 249–255. https://doi.org/10.1080/0142159X.2018.1543862

Howard, K. I., Mark, S., Merton, K., Krause, S., & Orlinsky, D. E. (1986). The dose-effect relationship in psychotherapy. *American Psychologist*, 41(2), 159–164. https://doi.org/10.1037/0003-066X.41.2.159

Huber, L., Gonzalez, T., Robles, G., & Solórzano, D. G. (2021). Racial microaffirmations as a response to racial microaggressions: Exploring risk and protective factors. *New Ideas in Psychology*, 63, 100880. https://doi.org/10.1016/j.newideapsych.2021.100880

Huber, L. P., Robles, G., & Solórzano, D. G. (2023). "Life was brought back into my body": a Critical Race Feminista analysis of racial microaffirmations. *Race Ethnicity and Education*, 26(6), 701–718. https://doi.org/10.1080/13613324.2023.2165514

Irving, G., Neves, A. L., Dambha-Miller, H., Oishi, A., Tagashira, H., Verho, A., & Holden, J. (2017). International variations in primary care physician consultation time: A systematic review of 67 countries. In *BMJ Open* (Vol. 7, Issue 10). BMJ Publishing Group. https://doi.org/10.1136/bmjopen-2017-017902

Jacobs, A. J. (2012). *Drop dead healthy: One man's humble quest for bodily perfection*. Simon & Schuster.

Jacobson, N. S., Christensen, A., Prince, S. E., Cordova, J., & Eldridge, K. (2000). Integrative behavioral couple therapy: An acceptance-based, promising new treatment for couple discord. *Journal of Consulting and Clinical Psychology*, 68(2), 351–355. https://doi.org/10.1037/0022

Jennissen, S., Huber, J., Ehrenthal, J. C., Schauenburg, H., & Dinger, U. (2018). Association between insight and outcome of psychotherapy: Systematic review and meta-analysis. *American Journal of Psychiatry*, 175(10), 961–969. https://doi.org/10.1176/appi.ajp.2018.17080847

Johnson, S. M. (2019). *Attachment theory in practice: Emotionally focused therapy (EFT) with individuals, couples, and families*. Guilford Publications.

Jones, J. M., Sander, J. B., & Booker, K. W. (2013). Multicultural competency building: Practical solutions for training and evaluating student progress. *Training and Education in Professional Psychology*, 7(1), 12–22. https://doi.org/10.1037/a0030880

Jung, C. G. (1960). *Synchronicity: An acausal connecting principle*. Princeton University Press.

Kahr, B. (2005). Letter from London: On Patients who remove their clothing. *American Imago*, 62(2), 217–223.

Kaslow, F. W. (2001). Whither countertransference in couples and family therapy: A systemic perspective. *Journal of Clinical Psychology*, 57(8), 1029–1040. https://doi.org/10.1002/jclp.1071

Khan, S., Faisal, K., & Rashid, A. (2022). KSAO based competency model for an effective practice of tele-counseling in Pakistan. *Journal of Professional & Applied Psychology*, 3(2), 276–292. https://doi.org/10.52053/jpap.v3i2.98

King Jr., M. L. (1965). *Remaining awake through a great revolution*. www2.ober lin.edu/external/EOG/BlackHistoryMonth/MLK/CommAddress.html

Kleespies, P. M., Penk, W. E., & Forsyth, J. P. (1993). The stress of patient suicidal behavior during clinical training: Incidence, impact, and recovery. *Professional Psychology: Research and Practice, 24*(3), 293–303.

Kleinplatz, P., & Ménard, A. D. (2020). *Magnificent sex*. Routledge.

Klettke, B., Hallford, D. J., & Mellor, D. J. (2014). Sexting prevalence and correlates: A systematic literature review. *Clinical Psychology Review, 34*(1), 44–53. https://doi.org/10.1016/j.cpr.2013.10.007

Koch, J. M., Knutson, D., Loche, L. T., Loche, R. W., Lee, H. S., & Federici, D. J. (2022). A qualitative inquiry of microaffirmation experiences among culturally diverse graduate students. *Current Psychology, 41*(5), 2883–2895. https://doi.org/10.1007/s12144-020-00811-3

Koval, C. Z., & Rosette, A. S. (2021). The natural hair bias in job recruitment. *Social Psychological and Personality Science, 12*(5), 741–750. https://doi.org/10.1177/1948550620937937

Krebs, P., Norcross, J. C., Nicholson, J. M., & Prochaska, J. O. (2018). Stages of change and psychotherapy outcomes: A review and meta-analysis. *Journal of Clinical Psychology, 74*(11), 1964–1979. https://doi.org/10.1002/jclp.22683

Kurdek, L. A. (2006). Differences between partners from heterosexual, gay, and lesbian cohabiting couples. *Journal of Marriage and Family, 68*(2), 509–528. https://doi.org/10.1111/j.1741-3737.2006.00268.x

Lamb, D. H., Catanzaro, S. J., & Moorman, A. S. (2003). Psychologists reflect on their sexual relationships with clients, supervisees, and students: Occurrence, impact, rationales, and collegial intervention. *Professional Psychology: Research and Practice, 34*(1), 102–107. https://doi.org/10.1037/0735-7028.34.1.102

Lambert, M. J. (2013). Outcome in psychotherapy: The past and important advances. *Psychotherapy, 50*(1), 42–51. https://doi.org/10.1037/a0030682

Lin, T., Stone, S. J., Heckman, T. G., & Anderson, T. (2021). Zoom-in to zoneout: Therapists report less therapeutic skill in telepsychology versus face-toface therapy during the COVID-19 pandemic. *Psychotherapy, 58*(4), 449–459. https://doi.org/10.1037/pst0000398

Linzer, M., Poplau, S., Babbott, S., Collins, T., Guzman-Corrales, L., Menk, J., Murphy, M. Lou, & Ovington, K. (2016). Worklife and wellness in academic general internal medicine: Results from a national survey. *Journal of General Internal Medicine, 31*(9), 1004–1010. https://doi.org/10.1007/s11606-016-3720-4

Littauer, H., Sexton, H., & Wynn, R. (2005). Qualities clients wish for in their therapists. *Scandinavian Journal of Caring Sciences, 19*(1), 28–31. https://doi.org/10.1111/j.1471-6712.2005.00315.x

McCluney, C. L., Durkee, M. I., Smith, R., Robotham, K. J., & Lee, S. S. L. (2021). To be, or not to be…Black: The effects of racial codeswitching on perceived professionalism in the workplace. *Journal of Experimental Social Psychology, 97*, 1–12. https://doi.org/10.1016/j.jesp.2021.104199

McDonald, D. N., Wantz, R. A., & Firmin, M. W. (2014). Sources informing undergraduate college student perceptions of psychologists. *Psychological Record, 64*, 537–542. https://doi.org/10.1007/s40732-014-0054-7

McGuinness, D., Dowling, M., & Trimble, T. (2013). Experiences of involuntary admission in an approved mental health centre. *Journal of Psychiatric and Mental Health Nursing, 20*(8), 726–734. https://doi.org/10.1111/jpm.12007

Meichenbaum, D., & Lilienfeld, S. O. (2018). How to spot hype in the field of psychotherapy: A 19-item checklist. *Professional Psychology: Research and Practice, 49*(1), 22–30. https://doi.org/10.1037/pro0000172

Meier, D., Tschacher, W., Frommer, A., Moggi, F., & Pfammatter, M. (2023). Growth curves of common factors in psychotherapy: Multilevel growth modelling and outcome analysis. *Clinical Psychology & Psychotherapy, 30*(5), 1095–1110. https://doi.org/10.1002/cpp.2864

Melamed, Y., Szor, H., & Berstein, E. (2001). The loneliness of the therapist in the public outpatient clinic. *Journal of Contemporary Psychotherapy, 31*, 103–112. https://doi.org/10.1023/A:1010213606443

Ménard, A. D., Bondy, M., Jones, M., Desjardins, L., Milidrag, L., Foulon, A., & Chittle, L. (2023). "I wasn't that good at it but I pretended to be": Students' experiences of the Impostor Phenomenon in academic settings. *Alberta Journal of Higher Education, 69*(3), 363–383. https://doi.org/10.11575/ajer.v69i3.76167

Ménard, A. D., & Chittle, L. (2023). The impostor phenomenon in post-secondary students: A review of the literature. *Review of Education, 11*(2), 1–32. https://doi.org/10.1002/rev3.3399

Ménard, A. D., Jaffri, S., Soucie, K., Cavallo-Medved, K., & Houser, C. (in press). Awareness, use and value of student support programs through the lens of science students, faculty and staff. *Canadian Journal for the Scholarship of Teaching and Learning.*

Ménard, A. D., Soucie, K., Jafri, S., Houser, C., & Cavallo-Medved, D. (2021). Concordance (or discordance) between students and staff/faculty perceptions of student stress in Science. *Canadian Journal for the Scholarship of Teaching and Learning, 12*(1). https://doi.org/10.5206/cjsotlrcacea.2021.1.10810

Miserandino, C. (2003). The spoon theory. Retrieved from https://butyoudontlooksick.com/articles/written-by-christine/the-spoon-theory/

Mosher, D. K., Hook, J. N., Captari, L. E., Davis, D. E., DeBlaere, C., & Owen, J. (2017). Cultural humility: A therapeutic framework for engaging diverse clients. *Practice Innovations, 2*(4), 221–233. https://doi.org/10.1037/pri0000055

Moss, J. (2019). Burnout is about your workplace, not your people. *Harvard Business Review.* Retrieved from https://hbr.org/2019/12/burnout-is-about-your-workplace-not-your-people

Nelson, M. L. (2014). Using the major formats of clinical supervision. In C. E. Watkins Jr. & D. L. Milne (Eds.), *The Wiley International Handbook of Clinical Supervision* (pp. 308–328). Wiley Blackwell.

Nelson, M. L., Barnes, K. L., Evans, A. L., & Triggiano, P. J. (2008). Working with conflict in clinical supervision: Wise supervisors' perspectives. *Journal of Counseling Psychology, 55*(2), 172–184. https://doi.org/10.1037/0022-0167.55.2.172.supp

Nelson, M. L., & Friedlander, M. L. (2001). A close look at conflictual supervisory relationships: The trainee's perspective. *Journal of Counseling Psychology, 48*(4), 384–395. https://doi.org/10.1037/0022-0167.48.4.384

Norcross, J. C. (2002). Empirically supported therapy relationships. In J. C. Norcross (Ed.), *Psychotherapy relationships that work: Therapist contributions and responsiveness to patients* (pp. 3–16), Oxford University Press.

Norcross, J. C., & Hill, C. E. (2004). Empirically supported therapy relationships. *The Clinical Psychologist, 57*(3), 19–24.

Norcross, J. C., & Lambert, M. J. (2018). Psychotherapy relationships that work III. *Psychotherapy, 55*(4), 303–315. https://doi.org/10.1037/pst0000193

O'Donovan, A., Halford, W. K., & Walters, B. (2011). Towards best practice supervision of clinical psychology trainees. *Australian Psychologist, 46*(2), 101–112. https://doi.org/10.1111/j.1742-9544.2011.00033.x

Olafsdottir, G., Cloke, P., Schulz, A., van Dyck, Z., Eysteinsson, T., Thorleifsdottir, B., & Vögele, C. (2020). Health benefits of walking in nature: A randomized controlled study under conditions of real-life stress. *Environment and Behavior, 52*(3), 248–274. https://doi.org/10.1177/0013916518800798

Opie, T. R., & Phillips, K. W. (2015). Hair penalties: the negative influence of Afrocentric hair on ratings of Black women's dominance and professionalism. *Frontiers in Psychology, 6*, 1–14. https://doi.org/10.3389/fpsyg.2015.01311

Oswalt, P. (2022). *Patton Oswalt: We all scream*. Netflix.

Owen, J., Tao, K. W., Imel, Z. E., Wampold, B. E., & Rodolfa, E. (2014). Addressing racial and ethnic microaggressions in therapy. *Professional Psychology: Research and Practice, 45*(4), 283–290. https://doi.org/10.1037/a0037420

Paris, J. (2023). *Fads and fallacies in psychiatry* (2nd ed.). Cambridge University Press.

Parker, S., Suetani, S., & Motamarri, B. (2017). On being supervised: getting value from a clinical supervisor and making the relationship work when it is not. *Australasian Psychiatry, 25*(6), 625–629. https://doi.org/10.1177/103985621 7734668

Peplau, L. A., & Fingerhut, A. W. (2007). The close relationships of Lesbians and Gay men. *Annual Review of Psychology, 58*, 405–424. https://doi.org/10.1146/annurev.psych.58.110405.085701

Pope, K. S., Keith-Spiegel, P., & Tabachnick, B. G. (1986). Sexual attraction to clients: The human therapist and the (sometimes) inhuman training system. *American Psychologist, 41*(2), 147–158. https://doi.org/10.1037/1931-3918.s.2.96

Posluns, K., & Gall, T. L. (2020). Dear mental health practitioners, take care of yourselves: A literature review on self-care. *International Journal for the Advancement of Counselling, 42*(1), 1–20. https://doi.org/10.1007/s10447-019-09382-w

Prochaska, J.O., & DiClemente, C.C. (1983). Stages and processes of self-change of smoking: toward an integrative model of change. *Journal of Consulting and Clinical Psychology, 51*(3), 390–395.

Richardson, C. M. E., Trusty, W. T., & George, K. A. (2020). Trainee wellness: self-critical perfectionism, self-compassion, depression, and burnout among doctoral trainees in psychology. *Counselling Psychology Quarterly, 33*(2), 187–198. https://doi.org/10.1080/09515070.2018.1509839

Rief, W., Kopp, M., Awarzamani, R., & Weise, C. (2022). Selected trends in psychotherapy research: An index analysis of RCTs. *Clinical Psychology in Europe*, 42(2), 1–15. https://doi.org/10.32872/cpe.7921

Rogers, C. (1951). *Client-centered therapy: Its current practice, implications, and theory*. Houghton Mifflin.

Rogers, C. (1961). *On becoming a person*. Houghton Mifflin.

Rowe, M. (2008). Micro-affirmations & micro-inequities. *Journal of the International Ombudsman Association*, 1(1), 45–48.

Sackett, C. R., Mack, H. L., Sharma, J., Cook, R. M., & Dogan-Dixon, J. (2023). A phenomenological exploration of counselors-in-Training's experiences of microaggressions from clients. *The Professional Counselor*, 13(2), 145–161. https://doi.org/10.15241/crs.13.2.145

Schwabe, L., & Wolf, O. T. (2010). Learning under stress impairs memory formation. *Neurobiology of Learning and Memory*, 93(2), 183–188. https://doi.org/10.1016/j.nlm.2009.09.009

Seidel, J. (2022, May 6). I swear, this is a bloody good study. *Cosmos Magazine*. Retrieved from https://cosmosmagazine.com/people/culture/australians-swearing/

Sharpless, B. A., & Barber, J. P. (2009). The Examination for Professional Practice in Psychology (EPPP) in the Era of Evidence-Based Practice. *Professional Psychology: Research and Practice*, 40(4), 333–340. https://doi.org/10.1037/a0013983

Sheaves, B., Isham, L., Bradley, J., Espie, C., Barrera, A., Waite, F., Harvey, A. G., Attard, C., & Freeman, D. (2018). Adapted CBT to stabilize sleep on psychiatric wards: A transdiagnostic treatment approach. *Behavioural and Cognitive Psychotherapy*, 46(6), 661–675. https://doi.org/10.1017/S1352465817000789

Silverstein, J. L. (1998). Counter transference in marital therapy for infidelity. *Journal of Sex and Marital Therapy*, 24(4), 293–301. https://doi.org/10.1080/00926239808403964

Smith, S. M., O'Kelly, S., & O'Dowd, T. (2010). GPs' and pharmacists' experiences of managing multimorbidity: A "Pandora's box." *British Journal of General Practice*, 60(576), e285–e295. https://doi.org/10.3399/bjgp10X514756

Snyder, C. M. J., & Anderson, S. A. (2009). An examination of mandated versus voluntary referral as a determinant of clinical outcome. *Journal of Marital and Family Therapy*, 35(3), 278–292. https://doi.org/10.1111/j.1752-0606.2009.00118.x

Snyder, D. K., & Halford, W. K. (2012). Evidence-based couple therapy: Current status and future directions. *Journal of Family Therapy*, 34(3), 229–249. https://doi.org/10.1111/j.1467-6427.2012.00599.x

Soares, E. E., Thrall, J. N., Stephens, T. N., Rodriguez Biglieri, R., Consoli, A. J., & Bunge, E. L. (2020). Publication trends in psychotherapy: Bibliometric analysis of the past 5 decades. *American Journal of Psychotherapy*, 73(3), 85–94. https://doi.org/10.1176/appi.psychotherapy.20190045

Spengler, E. S., Miller, D. J., & Spengler, P. M. (2016). Microaggressions: Clinical errors with sexual minority clients. *Psychotherapy*, 53(3), 360–366. https://doi.org/10.1037/pst0000073

Sprott, R. A., Herbitter, C., Grant, P., Moser, C., & Kleinplatz, P. J. (2023). Clinical guidelines for working with clients involved in kink. *Journal of Sex and Marital Therapy*. https://doi.org/10.1080/0092623X.2023.2232801

Sucala, M., Cuijpers, P., Muench, F., Cardoş, R., Soflau, R., Dobrean, A., ... & David, D. (2017). Anxiety: There is an app for that. A systematic review of anxiety apps. *Depression and Anxiety*, *34*(6), 518–525. https://doi.org/10.1002/da.22654

Sue, D. W., Alsaidi, S., Awad, M. N., Glaeser, E., Calle, C. Z., & Mendez, N. (2019). Disarming racial microaggressions: Microintervention strategies for targets, White allies, and bystanders. *American Psychologist*, *74*(1), 128. https://doi.org/10.1037/amp0000296

Tafrate, R. C., Mitchell, D., & Novaco, R. W. (2014). Forensic CBT: Five recommendations for clinical practice and five topics in need of more attention. In R. C. Tafrate & D. Mitchell (Eds.), *Forensic CBT: A handbook for clinical practice* (pp. 473–486). John Wiley & Sons, Ltd.

Talmi, A., Muther, E. F., Margolis, K., Buchholz, M., Asherin, R., & Bunik, M. (2016). The scope of behavioral health integration in a pediatric primary care setting. *Journal of Pediatric Psychology*, *41*(10), 1120–1132. https://doi.org/10.1093/jpepsy/jsw065

Tolin, D. (2016). *Doing CBT: A Comprehensive Guide to Working with Behaviors, Thoughts, and Emotions*. Guilford Press.

Twomey, M., Sammon, D., & Nagle, T. (2020). Memory recall/information retrieval challenges within the medical appointment: a review of the literature. *Journal of Decision Systems*, *29*(3), 148–181. https://doi.org/10.1080/12460125.2020.1809781

Vansteenwegen, A. (1998). Helpfulness of therapist verbal interventions in couple therapy. *Sexual and Marital Therapy*, *13*(1), 15–20. https://doi.org/10.1080/02674659808406540

Vesentini, L., Van Overmeire, R., Matthys, F., De Wachter, D., Van Puyenbroeck, H., & Bilsen, J. (2022). Intimacy in psychotherapy: An exploratory survey among therapists. *Archives of Sexual Behavior*, *51*(1), 453–463. https://doi.org/10.1007/s10508-021-02190-7

Vogel, D. L., Wester, S. R., & Larson, L. M. (2007). Avoidance of counseling: Psychological factors that inhibit seeking help. *Journal of Counseling and Development*, *85*(4), 410–422. https://doi.org/10.1002/j.1556-6678.2007.tb00609.x

Wahl, O., Reiss, M., & Thompson, C. A. (2018). Film psychotherapy in the 21st century. *Health Communication*, *33*(3), 238–245. https://doi.org/10.1080/10410236.2016.1255842

Wampold, B. E. (2015). How important are the common factors in psychotherapy? An update. *World Psychiatry*, *14*(3), 270–277. https://doi.org/10.1002/wps.20238

Watkins Jr., C. E. (2012). Educating psychotherapy supervisors. *American Journal of Psychotherapy*, *66*(3), 279–307.

Watkins Jr., C. E. (2017). How does psychotherapy supervision work? Contributions of connection, conception, allegiance, alignment, and action.

Journal of Psychotherapy Integration, 27(2), 201–217. https://doi.org/10.1037/int0000058

Watkins Jr., C. E., Reyna, S. H., Ramos, M. J., & Hook, J. N. (2015). The ruptured supervisory alliance and its repair: On supervisor apology as a reparative intervention. *Clinical Supervisor, 34*(1), 98–114. https://doi.org/10.1080/07325223.2015.1015194

Williams, I. L., & Uebel, M. (2021). On the use of profane language in psychotherapy and counseling: A brief summary of studies over the last six decades. *European Journal of Psychotherapy and Counselling, 23*(4), 404–421. https://doi.org/10.1080/13642537.2021.2001025

Winter, S., Diamond, M., Green, J., Karasic, D., Reed, T., Whittle, S., & Wylie, K. (2016). Transgender people: health at the margins of society. *The Lancet, 388*(10042), 390–400. https://doi.org/10.1016/S0140-6736(16)00683-8

Yalom, I. D. (2017). *The gift of therapy: An open letter to a new generation of therapists and their patients*. Harper Perennial.

Yalom, I. D., & Elkin, G. (1991). *Every day gets a little closer*. Basic Books.

Yourman, D. B. (2003). Trainee disclosure in psychotherapy supervision: The impact of shame. *Journal of Clinical Psychology, 59*(5), 601–609. https://doi.org/10.1002/jclp.10162

Ziede, J. S., & Norcross, J. C. (2020). Personal therapy and self-care in the making of psychologists. *Journal of Psychology: Interdisciplinary and Applied, 154*(8), 585–618. https://doi.org/10.1080/00223980.2020.1757596

Ziv-Beiman, S. (2013). Therapist self-disclosure as an integrative intervention. *Journal of Psychotherapy Integration, 23*(1), 59–74. https://doi.org/10.1037/a0031783

For Product Safety Concerns and Information please contact our EU
representative GPSR@taylorandfrancis.com
Taylor & Francis Verlag GmbH, Kaufingerstraße 24, 80331 München, Germany

www.ingramcontent.com/pod-product-compliance
Lightning Source LLC
Chambersburg PA
CBHW071103280326
41928CB00051B/2781